HANDBOOK OF PLACENTAL PATHOLOGY

Vijay V. Joshi, M.D., Ph.D., F.R.C.Path.
Professor and Director of Pediatric Pathology
and Clinical Professor of Pediatrics
East Carolina University School of Medicine
Greenville, North Carolina
and
Consultant in Pediatric Pathology
Beth Israel Medical Center
New York, New York

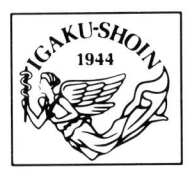

IGAKU-SHOIN   NEW YORK • TOKYO

Published and distributed by

IGAKU-SHOIN Medical Publishers, Inc.
One Madison Avenue, New York, New York 10010

IGAKU-SHOIN Ltd.,
5-24-3 Hongo, Bunkyo-ku, Tokyo 113-91.

Copyright © 1994 by IGAKU-SHOIN Medical Publishers, Inc.
All rights reserved. No part of this book may be translated or
reproduced in any form but by print, photo-print, microfilm or any
other means without written permission from the publisher.

Library of Congress Cataloging-in-Publication Data

Joshi, Vijay V., 1936–
    Handbook of placental pathology / Vijay V. Joshi.
      p.   cm.
    Includes bibliographical references and index.
    ISBN 0-89640-254-1. — ISBN 0-460-14254-2
    1. Placenta—Diseases. I. Title.
    [DNLM: 1. Placenta—pathology. 2. Placenta Diseases—pathology.
WQ 212 J83h 1994]
RG591.J67   1994
618.3'407—dc20
DNLM/DLC
for Library of Congress   93-46480
                                                                                                     CIP

ISBN: 0-89640-254-1   (New York)
ISBN: 4-260-14254-2   (Tokyo)

Printed and bound in the U.S.A.
10 9 8 7 6 5 4 3 2 1

HANDBOOK OF
PLACENTAL PATHOLOGY

PREFACE

The seeds of this book were sown when, about 4½ years ago, I started signing out placentas in large numbers for the first time in my career. In order to prepare for the task and approach it in a systematic manner, I started reading monographs, book chapters, and articles on the subject. I prepared a short write-up on placental pathology for my surgical pathologist colleagues. As I continued signing out placentas at the rate of about 1400 per year, and began seeing variants of common placental lesions and different types of uncommon and rare placental lesions, I felt the need to organize the process of signing out in a more systematic way. That led to the preparation of this handbook, which should serve as a concise yet comprehensive guide for general surgical pathologists in carrying out gross and microscopic examination of placentas and preparing reports systematically, expeditiously, and with better understanding of placental pathology. I believe that it should also be useful to trainees in pathology, obstetrics and gynecology, and neonatology, as well as to practicing clinicians in these specialties.

It is estimated that about 20% of the placentas from about 4 million births occurring every year in the United States are submitted to the surgical pathology laboratory. (It appears that in some countries, many of the placentas which are not sent to the surgical pathology laboratory are used for preparation of albumin, immunoglobulins, and collagen.) Thus pathologists working in all types of hospitals are likely to get placentas in their laboratories. The single-author and multiauthor monographs on placental pathology published in the past several years are excellent and comprehensive. However, they are not oriented to the needs of busy surgical pathologists, clinicians, and trainees in various specialties. On the other hand, the chapters on placental pathology in various textbooks of pathology and its subspecialties are not sufficiently comprehensive for their needs. This handbook occupies an intermediate position. In the opening section of the book, the normal structure of the placenta is briefly described. Common gross and microscopic lesions of the placenta are briefly discussed and adequately illustrated. These sections will help both the trainee and the practicing physician to develop a better understanding of and a systematic approach to placental pathology. The subsequent sections describe and illustrate the primary lesions of the placenta, as well as those lesions seen in maternal and fetal disorders. Besides the pathologic features, pathogenesis and clinical significance are described in every section for better understanding of various lesions. Tables which summarize the features of various lesions are suited for quick reference by the side of the microscope while one is signing out a case. In addition, pertinent original and recent references are cited at the end of the book. These references should serve as the source of more detailed discussion of various topics. Those who wish to keep up with the literature on the placenta need to review not only pathology journals but also obstetrics journals and the journal *Placenta*. This book, which represents an attempt to fulfill the practical needs of practicing and trainee physicians, is largely based on material which has been published by various investigators. However, wherever indicated, I have given my own views and related my own experience. I hope that the readers will find the book helpful.

Vijay V. Joshi, M.D., Ph.D., F.R.C.Path.
Greenville, NC

DEDICATION

Dedicated with love, respect, and gratitude to the memory of my late father, Baba, who passed away during the preparation of this book.

ACKNOWLEDGMENT

I am indebted to many individuals. I would like to mention particularly my cousin, Dr. Vasant (Chachan) G. Joshi who was my role model during my medical school years and postgraduate training. My teachers and mentors have provided guidance from the beginning of my career and during my formative years as a pediatric pathologist. My surgical pathologist colleagues at the East Carolina University of Medicine have provided encouragement. Professor H. Thomas Norris and Dean James Hallock have provided unstinting support and an appreciation of my efforts. Dr. Alexander Knisely and Dr. Shyan Sun have provided three of the photographs included in this book. The credit for taking the gross photographs goes to the team of pathologists' assistants headed by Mr. John Mitchell. Mr. John Artois and his staff devoted a great deal of effort and expertise to the preparation of the photographs for publication. Mr. Alan Branigan and his staff used their artistic talents in preparing the diagrams. Ms. Pauline Hardee, Ms. Tricia Robbins, and Ms. Dee Mullins typed numerous drafts of the various sections of the book. Ms. Lila Maron and the production staff of Igaku-Shoin provided support during the preparation of the book. I express my sincere thanks to all of these individuals, who have acted as teachers, mentors, helpful colleagues, and coworkers. Last, but not least, my wife, Jayashree, and our sons, Abhijit and Jitendra, have shown patience and understanding and have given their full cooperation while I was preparing this book.

Vijay V. Joshi, M.D., Ph.D., F.R.C.Path.

CONTENTS

INTRODUCTION	1
DEVELOPMENT OF THE PLACENTA	2
STRUCTURE OF THE PLACENTA	2
Fibrin (Fibrinoid) in the Placenta	7
EXAMINATION OF THE PLACENTA IN THE CLINICAL SETTING	12
CLINICAL DATA TO BE SENT TO THE PATHOLOGIST	13
INDICATIONS FOR PATHOLOGIC EXAMINATION	14
PATHOLOGIC EXAMINATION OF THE PLACENTA	14
Gross Examination	15
Sections for Histologic Examination	16
Surgical Pathology Report	22
Retention of the Specimen	22
GROSS ABNORMALITIES OF THE PLACENTA	22
Lesions Due to Disturbances of Maternal Blood Flow	22
Perivillous Fibrin	22
Subchorionic Fibrin	24
Subchorial Thrombosis (Brues' Mole)	24
Retroplacental Hematoma (RH)	25
Marginal Hematoma	28
Placental Infarct	28
Lesions Due to Disturbance of Fetal Blood Flow	29
Intervillous Thrombus	29
Kline's Hemorrhage	29
Fetal Artery Thrombosis	30
Subamniotic Hematoma	30

Noncirculatory Lesions	**30**
Calcification	30
Chorionic Cysts	31

HISTOLOGIC LESIONS OF THE PLACENTA — 32

Lesions of the Villi Involving Trophoblast	**32**
Excessive Number of Syncytiotrophoblastic Knots	32
Excessive Number of Cytotrophoblastic Cells	33
Deficiency of Vasculosyncytial Membranes	34
Fibrinoid Necrosis of Villi (Intravillous Fibrinoid)	34
Lesions of Villi Involving Trophoblastic Basement Membrane	**34**
Lesions of Villi Involving Stroma	**35**
Stromal Fibrosis	35
Villous Edema	35
Abnormalities of Villous Blood Vessels	**36**
Generalized Abnormalities of Villi	**36**
Lesions Involving Fetal Stem Arteries	**37**
Fibromuscular Sclerosis	37
Obliterative Endarteritis	37
Hemorrhagic Endovasculitis (HEV)	38
Histopathology of Maternal Uteroplacental Arteries	**38**

LESIONS OF THE PLACENTA AS A WHOLE OR OF THE PLACENTAL DISK — 41

Large Placenta	**41**
Small Placenta	**42**
Extrachorial Placentas	**42**
Placenta Membranacea	**43**
Bilobate Placenta	**43**
Accessory or Succenturiate Lobe	**43**
Placenta Previa	**43**
Placenta Accreta	**44**
Retroplacental Hematoma (RH) and Abruptio Placentae (AP)	**45**
Maternal Floor Infarction	**45**
Villitis	**46**

Chronic Intervillositis	48
Bacterial Villitis	49
Viral Villitis	51
Human Immunodeficiency Virus (HIV) Infection	54
Fungal Infection	56
Parasitic Infection	56
Villitis of Unknown Etiology	57
Tumors of the Placenta	**58**
Hemangioma	59
Teratoma	59
Metastatic Tumors	60

LESIONS OF THE UMBILICAL CORD — 60

Short and Long Umbilical Cords	**61**
Single Umbilical Artery (SUA)	61
Supernumerary Umbilical Vessels	61
Varices and Aneurysms	61
Thrombosis of Umbilical Blood Vessels	**62**
Hematoma and Rupture of Umbilical Blood Vessels	**62**
Calcification of Umbilical Blood Vessels	**63**
Abnormal Insertion of the Umbilical Cord	**63**
Knots in the Umbilical Cord	**63**
Torsion of the Umbilical Cord	**64**
Stricture of the Umbilical Cord	**64**
Edema of the Umbilical Cord	**65**
Embryonic Remnants of the Umbilical Cord	**66**
Cysts of the Umbilical Cord	**66**
Tumors of the Umbilical Cord	**66**
Prolapse of the Umbilical Cord	**67**
Entanglement of the Umbilical Cord	**67**
Umbilical Vasculitis and Funisitis	**67**

LESIONS OF THE MEMBRANES — 67

Squamous Metaplasia	**68**
Amnion Nodosum	**68**

Amniotic Cysts, Rests, and Polyps	**69**
Amniotic Web	**69**
Amniotic Band Syndrome (ABS)	**70**
Extramembranous Pregnancy	**71**
Extraamniotic Pregnancy	**72**
Meconium Staining of the Membranes	**72**
Significance of Meconium	72
Time Interval Between Meconium Passage and Birth	73
Pathologic Features of Meconium Staining	73
Acute Chorioamnionitis (ACA)	**75**
Definition	75
Etiology	76
Clinical Significance	78
Chronic Chorioamnionitis (CCA)	**80**
Funisitis	**80**
Amniotic Fluid Embolism (AME)	**80**
Tumors of Placental Membranes	**81**
ABNORMALITIES OF THE DECIDUA	**81**
Terminology	**81**
Deciduitis	**81**
Decidual Vasculopathy	**81**
LESIONS OF THE PLACENTA IN MATERNAL DISORDERS	**81**
Toxemia of Pregnancy	**81**
Gross Features	81
Histologic Features	82
Pathogenesis	82
Comment	83
Maternal Hypertension	**84**
Maternal Diabetes	**84**
Gross Features	84
Histologic Features	84
Pathogenesis	84
Comment	84

Abortion	**88**
Gross Features	88
Histologic Features	88
Pathogenesis	89
Comment	89
Premature Labor and Delivery	**89**
Gross Features	89
Histologic Features	89
Pathogenesis	89
Comment	89
Postmaturity	**90**
Gross Features	90
Histologic Features	90
Pathogenesis	90
Oligohydramnios and Polyhydramnios	**90**
Premature, Preterm, and Prolonged Rupture of Membranes	**91**
Maternal Fever	**91**
Maternal Substance Abuse	**91**
Abruptio Placentae	92
Systemic Lupus Erythematosus (SLE), Lupus Anticoagulant, and Anticardiolipin	92
LESIONS OF THE PLACENTA IN FETAL DISORDERS	**92**
Multiple Births	**92**
Twin Births	92
Demonstration of Vascular Anastomoses	98
Histologic Features	101
Types of Placentas in Twin Pregnancy	**104**
Monochorionic Diamniotic (MoDi) Placenta	104
Dichorionic Diamniotic (DiDi) Placenta	106
Monochorionic Monoamniotic (MoMo) Placenta	106
Vanishing Twins (VT)	107
Fetus Papyraceus/Fetus Compressus (FP/FC)	107
Acardiac Twins	107
Conjoined Twins (Siamese Twins)	108
Triplet and Multiple Births	108

Intrauterine Growth Retardation (IUGR)	109
Erythroblastosis Fetalis (EF)	109
Placenta in Nonimmunologic Hydrops Fetalis	110
Chromosomal Disorders	110
Metabolic Disorders	110
Antepartum Intrauterine Death with Retention and Maceration of the Fetus	111
Intrapartum Fetal Death	112
IATROGENIC LESIONS OF THE PLACENTA, UMBILICAL CORD, AND MEMBRANES	112
TRAUMATIC LESIONS OF THE PLACENTA	113
PLACENTA IN PREGNANCIES AFTER IN VITRO FERTILIZATION (IVF) AND EMBRYO TRANSFER (ET)	113
SPECIMENS RELATED TO PLACENTAL LASER SURGERY	113
COMMENT	114
INDEX	123

TABLES AND APPENDIX

Table 1 Types of Villi and Their Structure	17
Table 2 Histologic Assessment of Placenta	20
Table 3 Basic Gross Lesions of Placenta	24
Table 4 Basic Histologic Lesions of the Placenta	32
Table 5 Normal Range of Gross and Microscopic Lesions of the Term Placenta	41
Table 6 Weights of Placenta at Various Gestational Ages	42
Table 7 Salient Features of the Placenta in Maternal Disorders	85
Table 8 Classification of Diabetes Mellitus in Pregnancy	88
Table 9 Salient Features of Placenta in Fetal Disorders	93
Table 10 Ultrasonographic Criteria for Twin Transfusion Syndrome	105
Table 11 Neonatal Criteria for Twin Transfusion Syndrome	105

APPENDIX 1

Format of Reporting Gross and Microscopic Findings of Placenta	23

PATHOLOGY OF THE PLACENTA

INTRODUCTION

The placenta (the term derived from Latin that translates as "flat cake") provides oxygen, nourishment, and protection to the fetus. It also has excretory and endocrine functions. Numerous hormones such as human chorionic gonadotropin, progesterone, estrone, estradiol, estriol, and human placental lactogen are secreted by the placenta. Thus the trophoblast contributes significantly to the hormonal milieu during pregnancy. Examination of the placenta in the cases of poor pregnancy outcome and certain maternal disorders provides proper documentation and information useful to the obstetrician and neonatologist. Pathologic lesions of the placenta can be broadly classified into three types depending on their clinical relevance: (1) lesions responsible for fetal or neonatal morbidity and mortality (infarction, infection, abruption, etc.), (2) lesions related to premature expulsion of the fetus (chorioamnionitis, retroplacental hemorrhage, etc.), and (3) lesions that are likely to modify immediate clinical management of the mother (e.g., hydatidiform mole).

The placenta has not been a particularly favorite subject of the surgical pathologists for the following reasons.[1,2] There are too many of them (4 million births per year in the United States), the terminology is different from the usual surgical pathology terminology, the yield of information is low, and whatever information is obtained is unlikely to be unexpected and to have an immediate and direct clinical impact or significance. Further, interpretation of findings is difficult because there is an overlap between the findings in the normal and abnormal placenta, and quantitative studies that can be applied in practice are generally lacking. There are also the questions of who bears the cost of placental examination and of reducing the cost of medical care. However, the results of placental examination in certain cases do explain perinatal morbidity or mortality and have an impact on management of the mother and/or infant.

In recent years there have been new reasons for taking the placental examination more seriously. There has been an increase in malpractice suits against obstetricians. An American College of Obstetrics and Gynecology survey revealed that 73% of its fellows were sued at least once.[3] In some cases, the placental pathologic findings have indicated that the cause of the infant's difficulty antedated the delivery. The defendant's pathologist explains abnormal placental findings (extensive infarction, anomalous cord insertion, chorioamnionitis, villitis, etc.) that were related to the poor pregnancy outcome. As a result of the placental findings, juries have found physicians to be not liable for negligence or for causation of the poor outcome of pregnancy.

In 1989 the College of American Pathologists convened a conference entitled "Examination of Placenta: Patient Care and Risk Management." Pathologists with expertise in placental pathology, obstetricians, neonatologists, and attorneys were invited to participate. The proceedings were published in the July 1991 issue of *Archives of Pathology and Laboratory Medicine*. The articles in that issue have been consulted extensively in this book (the articles are referenced specifically in the text). The other major sources of information for this book are the three monographs on placental pathology by Fox, Benirschke and Kauffman, and Perrin[4-6] and personal experience. Neoplastic lesions of the trophoblast are not considered in this discussion.

DEVELOPMENT OF THE PLACENTA

After repeated mitotic divisions, the zygote, composed of the fused male and female pronuclei, transforms into a multicellular (12–16 cells) morula. A fluid-filled cavity appears in the morula to form a blastocyst. The outer layer of the blastocyst is the trophoblast (Gr., *trophe* = nutrition), and the inner cell mass is the embryoblast. The blastocyst attaches to the endometrium 6 days after fertilization. The trophoblast proliferates and differentiates into the outer syncytiotrophoblast and the inner cytotrophoblast. Invasion of the endometrium by the trophoblast enables the embryo to implant into and derive nourishment from the endometrium. A small space, the amniotic cavity, appears between the embryoblast and the trophoblast. Amnioblasts derived from the cytotrophoblast line this cavity and form the amnion. Lacunae that appear in the proliferating trophoblast become filled with maternal blood. This represents the beginning of the uteroplacental circulation. The maternal blood returns to the maternal circulation via the maternal veins. Fusion of adjacent lacunae results in the formation of lacunar networks, which are the primitive intervillous spaces. The cytotrophoblastic proliferation leads to the formation of small localized masses or primitive villi extending into the syncytiotrophoblast. These primitive villi and the extraembryonic somatic mesoderm constitute the chorion. The chorion forms the chorionic sac. The embryo and the amniotic sac are suspended within it by a connecting stalk that eventually develops into the umbilical cord. The connecting stalk contains the allantois, two arteries, and two veins. At later stages the right umbilical vein disappears. Up to about the 8th week, the chorionic villi cover the entire surface of the chorionic sac. With the growth of the sac there is compression atrophy of the villi along the decidua capsularis. Thus the chorion laeve or smooth chorion is formed. The villi along the decidua basalis rapidly proliferate, resulting in the formation of the chorionic plate and villous chorion (chorion frondosum). The amniotic sac increases in size at a faster rate than the chorionic sac. Therefore, there is fusion of the amnion and smooth chorion, with the formation of the amniochorionic membrane. The membrane fuses with the decidua capsularis and eventually with the decidua parietalis (Figure 1).

STRUCTURE OF THE PLACENTA

On gross examination the placenta consists of (1) the placental disk, (2) the extraplacental membranes, and (3) the umbilical cord (Figures 2 and 3). The

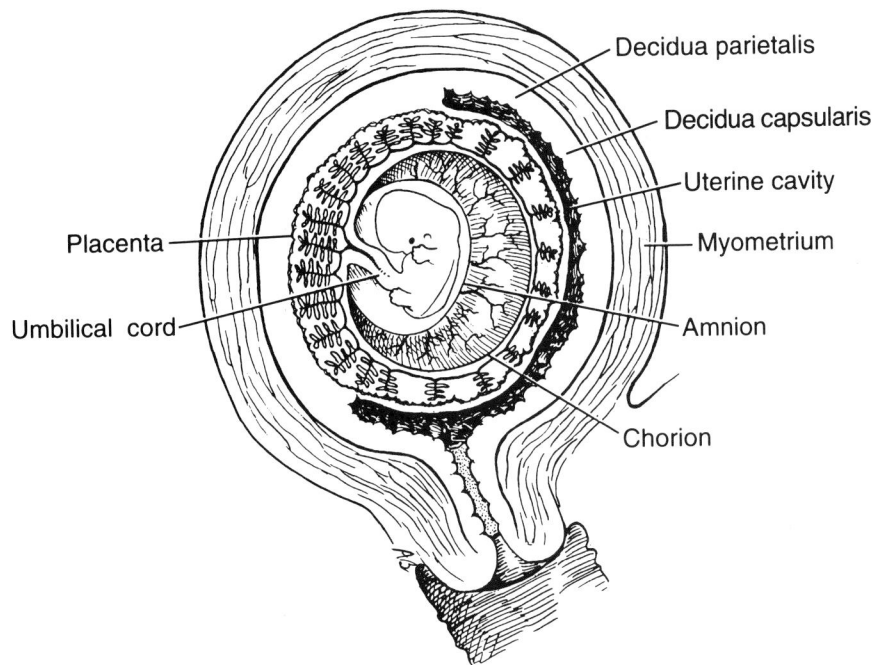

FIGURE 1. Diagrammatic representation of the gravid uterus with the placenta and the fetus.

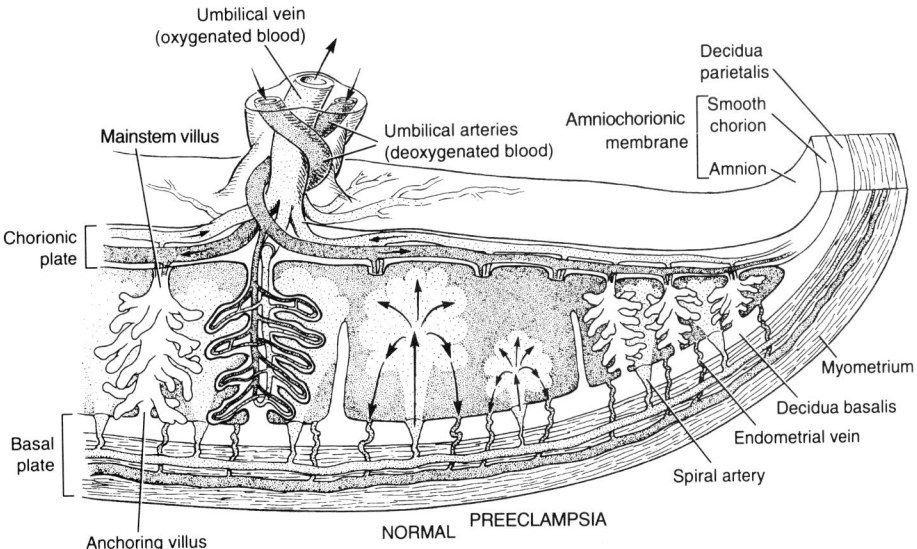

FIGURE 2. Diagrammatic representation of the structure of the placenta showing the fetal and maternal blood circulation through the placenta, ramifications of the villi, and chorionic and basal plates. (Adapted from Moore KL: *The developing human: Clinically oriented embryology.* WB Saunders Co., Philadelphia, 1988, Chap 7, Figure 7.6)

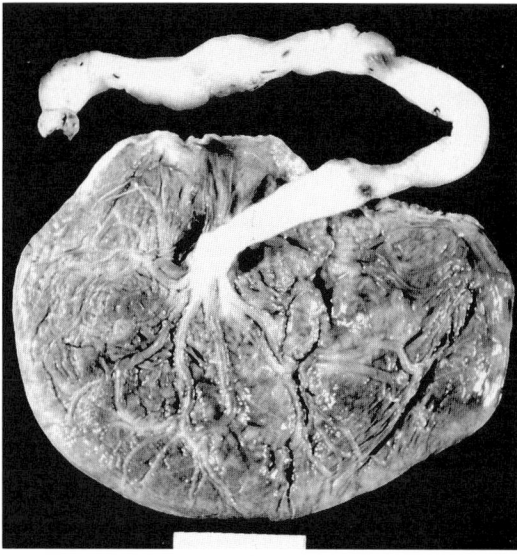

FIGURE 3. Fetal surface of the placenta. Note the insertion of the umbilical cord and the arteries and veins coursing along the fetal surface.

placental disk has the chorionic plate at the fetal surface and the cotyledons and basal plate at the maternal surface. The fetal surface, i.e., the chorionic plate, is covered with the amnion, and the cord is inserted normally on the fetal surface. The free membranes are normally inserted at the margin of the placental disk (Figures 3, 4).

On microscopic examination the following structures are noted:

1. *Placental disk*
    a. *Chorionic plate*: amnion, chorion, subchorionic fibrin, branches of umbilical blood vessels coursing along the stem villi (Figure 5).

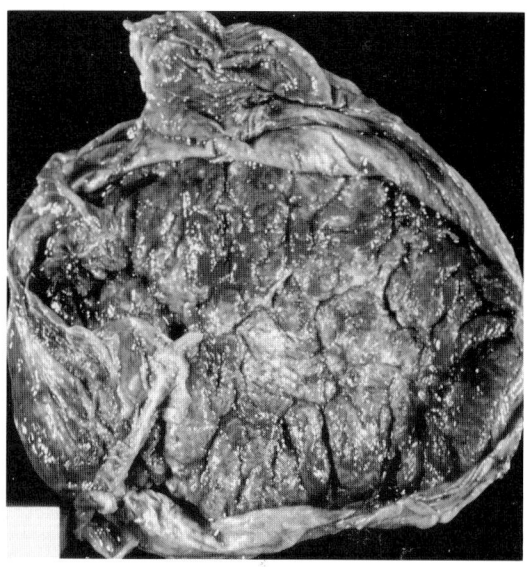

FIGURE 4. Maternal surface of the placenta (gross). Note the intact cotyledons and the marginally inserted membranes. The grooves separate the cotyledons.

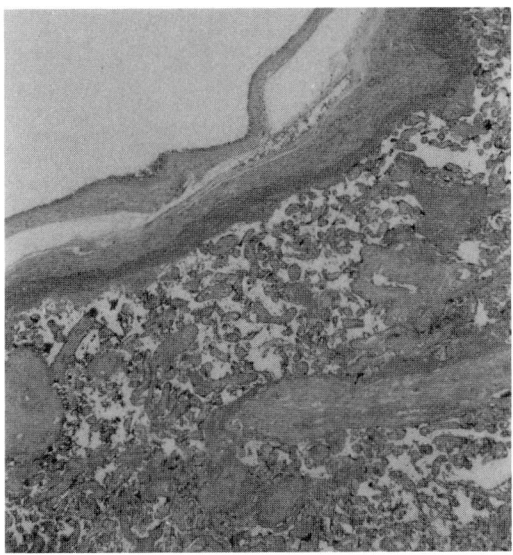

FIGURE 5. Note the amnion covering the chorionic plate, branches of umbilical blood vessels in the chorion, thin layer of subchorionic fibrin, and stem villi carrying the larger branches of umbilical blood vessels (H&E, ×40).

b. *Placental parenchyma:* stem, intermediate and terminal villi, intervillous space (Figures 6 to 8).
c. *Placental septa and extravillous trophoblastic cell islands.* During embryogenesis most of the trophoblast is used in the development of the villi. The remaining trophoblast, called "extravillous trophoblast," is used in the formation of other chorionic parts of the placenta, i.e., the chorionic plate, chorion laeve, septa, and cell islands. The septa arising from the basal plate subdivide the placenta into cotyledons (intercotyledonary

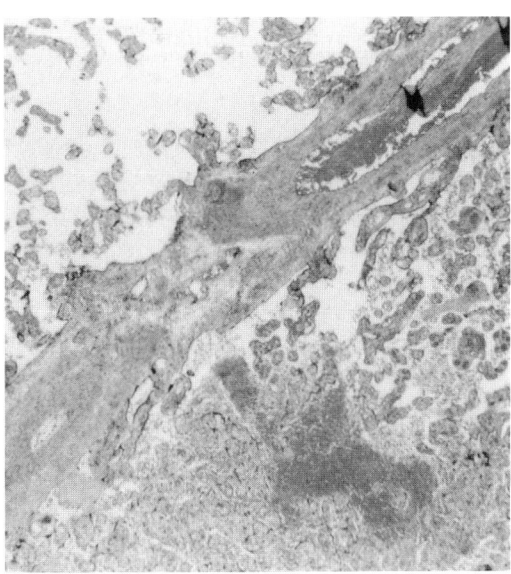

FIGURE 6. Stem villus with larger placental blood vessels that are branches of umbilical blood vessels (H&E, ×40).

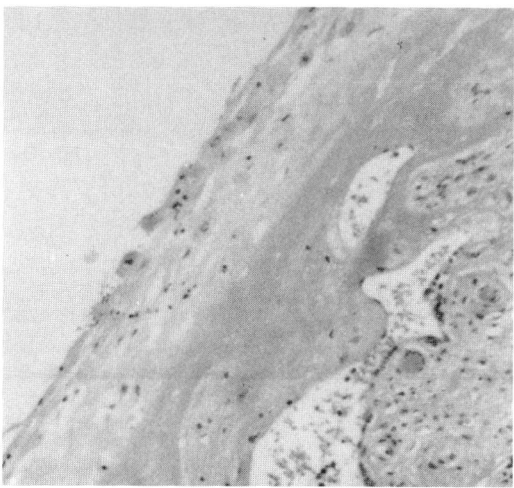

FIGURE 11. Basal plate of the placenta composed of the decidua basalis, fibrinoid, and extravillous trophoblastic cells. Note also the anchoring villus (H&E, ×250).

ical supporting framework in the placenta and also as an immunologic barrier protecting the fetus and placenta from the maternal immunologic reaction.

The term "fibrin" generally refers to the lamellar precipitates of fibrin in the blood vessels. "Fibrinoid" is a nonfibrous, noncellular, and more or less homogeneous product of the placenta. It may be a product of a combination of cellular secretion, cellular degeneration, and blood clotting. Fibrinoid is composed of fibrin with the addition of hyaluronic acid, sialic acid, immunoglobulins, albumin, etc. The terms "fibrin" and "fibrinoid" are used interchangeably or are considered to have different connotations. It has been suggested that the term "fibrinoid" be used when the exclusive derivation of the material as a product of blood clotting cannot be confirmed. Others have recommended the general use of the term "fibrinoid." In this chapter the term "fibrin" is used in

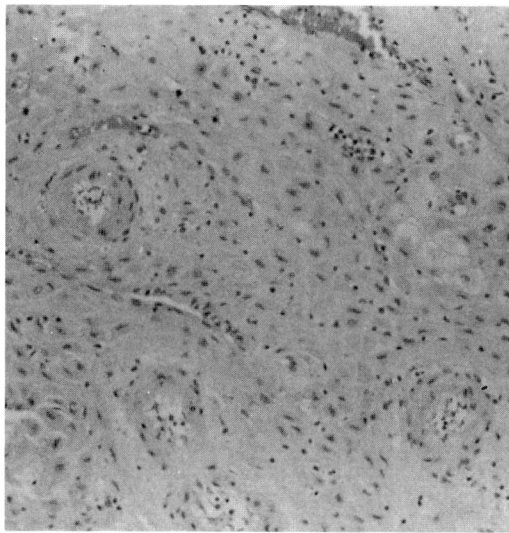

FIGURE 12. Normal maternal arteries in the decidua basalis.

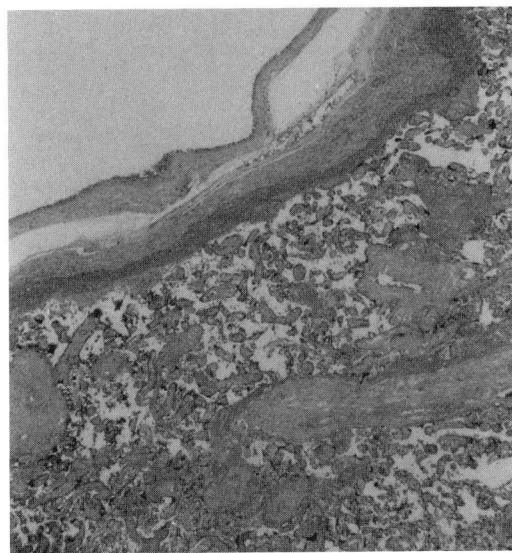

FIGURE 5. Note the amnion covering the chorionic plate, branches of umbilical blood vessels in the chorion, thin layer of subchorionic fibrin, and stem villi carrying the larger branches of umbilical blood vessels (H&E, ×40).

    b. *Placental parenchyma*: stem, intermediate and terminal villi, intervillous space (Figures 6 to 8).
    c. *Placental septa and extravillous trophoblastic cell islands.* During embryogenesis most of the trophoblast is used in the development of the villi. The remaining trophoblast, called "extravillous trophoblast," is used in the formation of other chorionic parts of the placenta, i.e., the chorionic plate, chorion laeve, septa, and cell islands. The septa arising from the basal plate subdivide the placenta into cotyledons (intercotyledonary

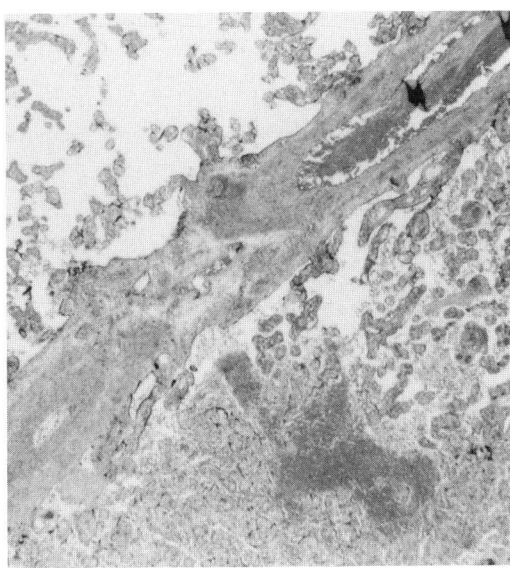

FIGURE 6. Stem villus with larger placental blood vessels that are branches of umbilical blood vessels (H&E, ×40).

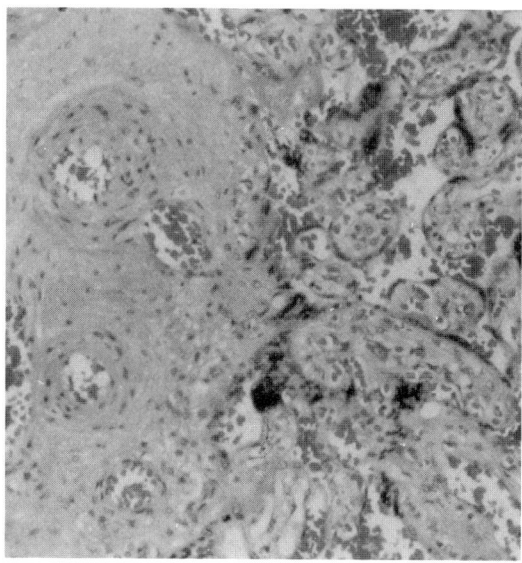

FIGURE 7. Stem villus and terminal villi. Note the cross section of normal placental arteries and veins. There are also terminal villi showing a syncytiotrophoblast with syncytial knots, villous capillaries, and stroma (H&E, ×100).

septa) (Figure 9). The grooves on the maternal surface are indicative of their position (Figure 4). The septa are incomplete, i.e., rarely reach the fetal surface. Extravillous trophoblasts, i.e., X cells, and a few decidual cells are present in the septa. The cell islands are connected to the villous tree or the chorionic plate (Figure 10). Cell islands are composed primarily of extravillous trophoblast. A small number of decidual cells may be present. Septa and cell islands also contain fibrinoid material.

d. *Basal plate:* fibrin, extravillous trophoblastic cells, decidua basalis, and maternal blood vessels (Figures 11 and 12).

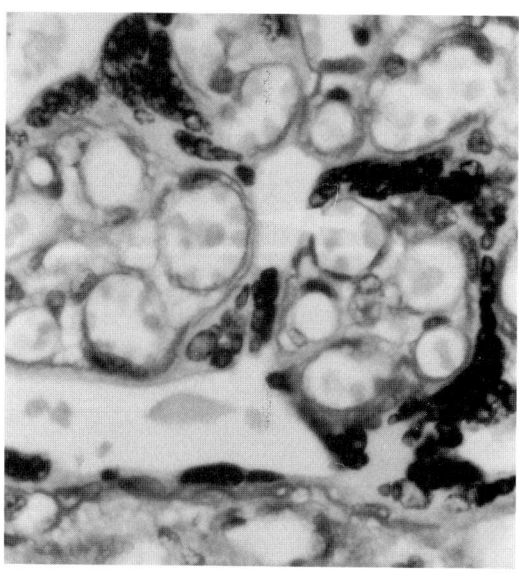

FIGURE 8. Terminal villi. Note the numerous (up to five) capillaries with little intervening stroma, trophoblastic basement membrane, vasculosyncytial membrane, and syncytiotrophoblast with syncytial knots (PAS, ×400).

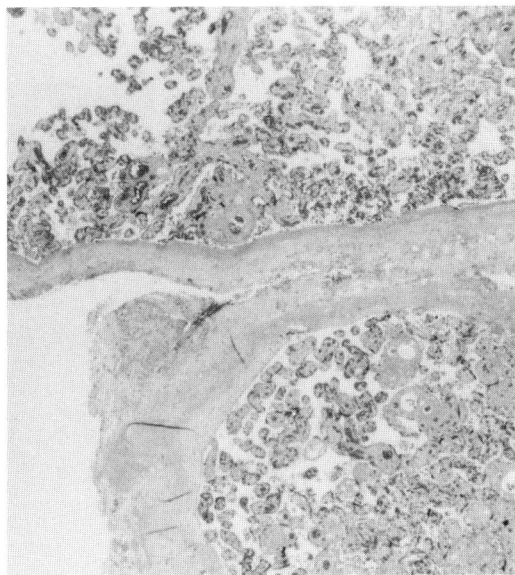

FIGURE 9. Placental septum arising from the maternal surface. There are two cotyledons in the figure (one on either side of the septum). The septum is composed of decidual cells, fibrinoid, and extravillous trophoblast.

2. *Membranes.* amniotic epithelium and connective tissue, potential space, chorion composed of extravillous trophoblastic cells and involuted villi (Figure 13), attached decidua capsularis and parietalis, maternal blood vessels, and remnant of the yolk sac seen as a yellowish white, firm, oval, slightly raised nodule measuring a few millimeters in diameter, usually near the insertion of the umbilical cord (Figure 14).
3. *Cord.* Surface epithelium, two arteries, one vein, and Wharton's jelly.

Fibrin (Fibrinoid) in the Placenta

Fibrinoid is one of the most prominent substances one sees during the gross and microscopic examination of the placenta. Fibrinoid may serve as a mechan-

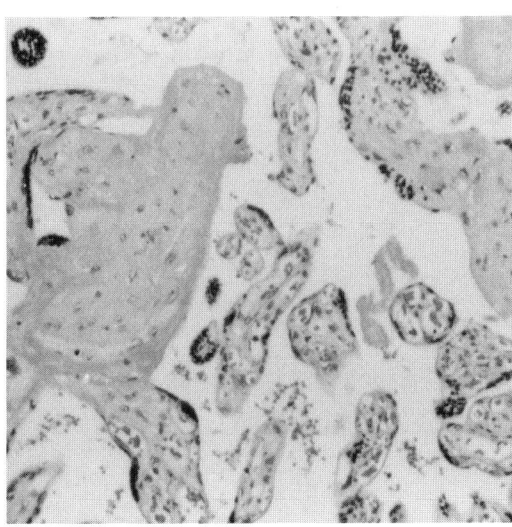

FIGURE 10. Cell island composed of extravillous trophoblast and fibrinoid material (H&E, ×100).

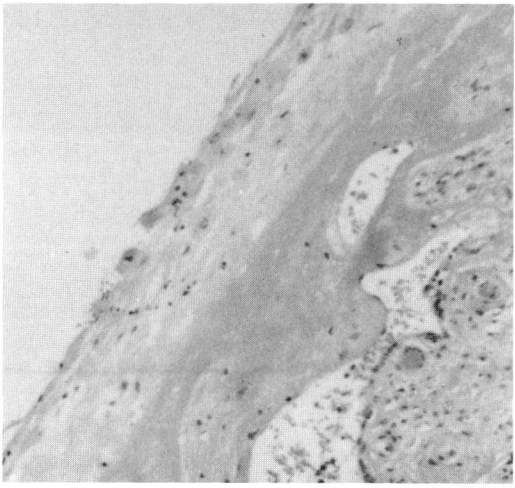

FIGURE 11. Basal plate of the placenta composed of the decidua basalis, fibrinoid, and extravillous trophoblastic cells. Note also the anchoring villus (H&E, ×250).

ical supporting framework in the placenta and also as an immunologic barrier protecting the fetus and placenta from the maternal immunologic reaction.

The term "fibrin" generally refers to the lamellar precipitates of fibrin in the blood vessels. "Fibrinoid" is a nonfibrous, noncellular, and more or less homogeneous product of the placenta. It may be a product of a combination of cellular secretion, cellular degeneration, and blood clotting. Fibrinoid is composed of fibrin with the addition of hyaluronic acid, sialic acid, immunoglobulins, albumin, etc. The terms "fibrin" and "fibrinoid" are used interchangeably or are considered to have different connotations. It has been suggested that the term "fibrinoid" be used when the exclusive derivation of the material as a product of blood clotting cannot be confirmed. Others have recommended the general use of the term "fibrinoid." In this chapter the term "fibrin" is used in

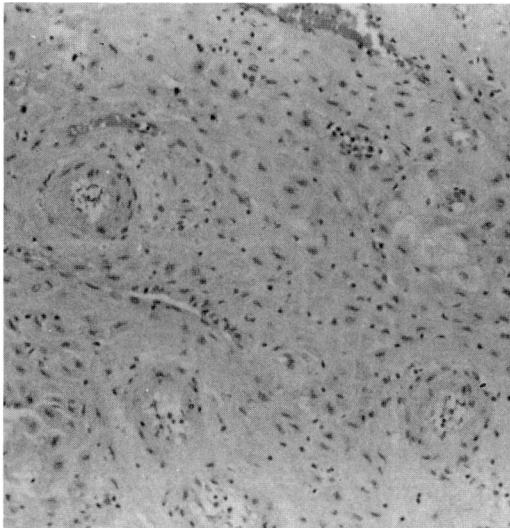

FIGURE 12. Normal maternal arteries in the decidua basalis.

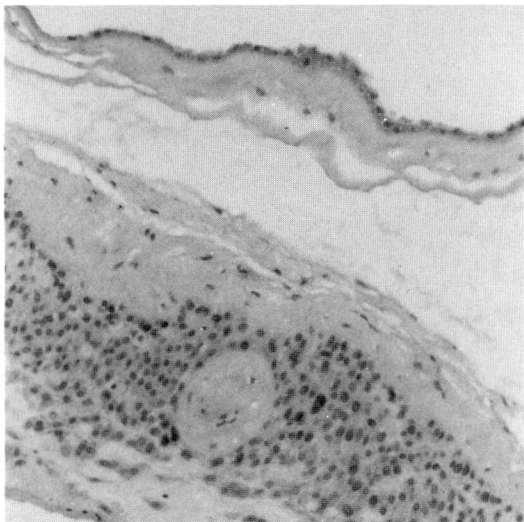

FIGURE 13. Normal membranes composed of amnion and chorion. Note the epithelium, connective tissue of the amnion and the atrophic villus, extravillous trophoblast, and connective tissue of the chorion (H&E, ×100).

reference to the material derived from blood clotting (e.g., subchorionic fibrin, perivillous fibrin). However, when the derivation is not clear, the term "fibrinoid" is used (e.g., intravillous fibrinoid or fibrinoid necrosis of villi, fibrinoid change in the media of maternal arteries).

The following localizations of the fibrin and/or fibrinoid are seen in both the normal and abnormal placenta (in abnormal placentas, fibrin and/or fibrinoid may be present in excessive amounts):

1. *Subchorionic fibrin (Langhans' stria) at the inferior surface of the chorionic plate.* This appears as whitish, firm plaques when viewed from the fetal surface and laminated material on the cut surface and also on histologic

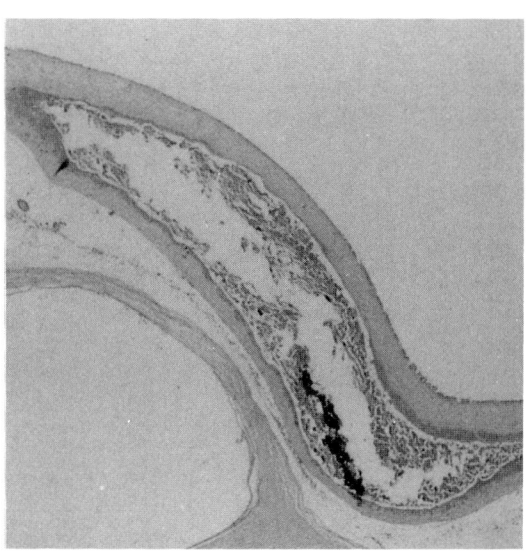

FIGURE 14. Remnant of the yolk sac on the fetal surface. Note the calcification (H&E, ×40).

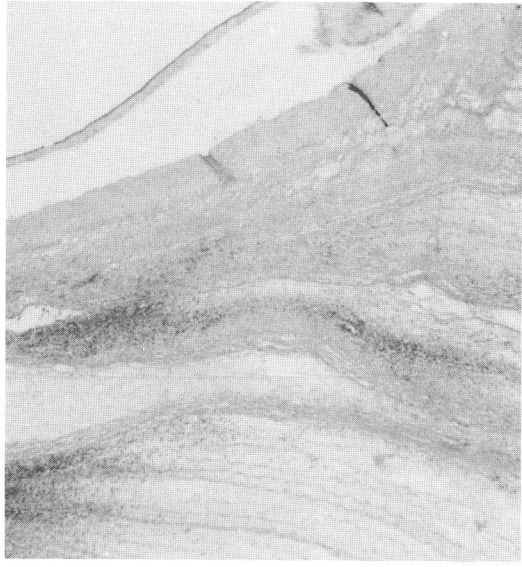

FIGURE 15. Subchorionic fibrin deposition.

examination (Figure 15). It is seen in about 20% of term placentas.[4] The fibrin deposition is related to turbulence and stasis of the maternal blood flow as it changes direction in the subchorionic zone. A moderate amount of subchorionic fibrin is of no clinical significance.

2. *Perivillous fibrin.* This is seen on gross examination in about 22% of the term placentas[7] and on histologic examination in all placentas (Figure 16). The foci vary from a few hundred micrometers to a few millimeters. Individual villi are trapped in fibrin. In the early stage the trapped villi may appear normal (Figure 16). Later they show degeneration and loss of syncytiotrophoblast followed by stromal fibrosis and hypovascularity (Figure 17). Perivil-

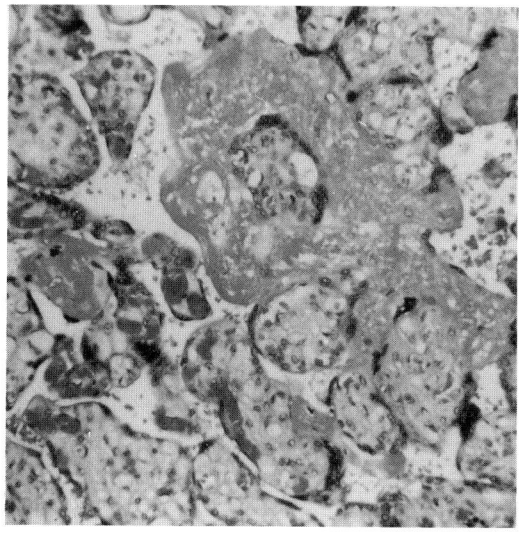

FIGURE 16. Perivillous fibrin deposition; in the early stage the trapped villus appears normal (H&E, ×100).

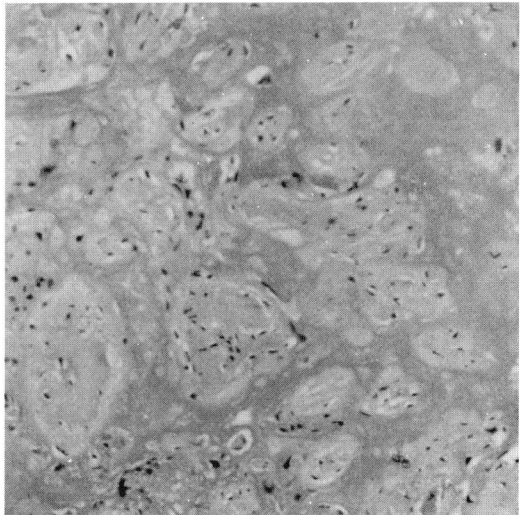

FIGURE 17. Perivillous fibrin deposition. Note the absence of syncytiotrophoblast in the trapped villi, which also show stromal fibrosis (H&E, ×100).

lous fibrin represents thrombosis of maternal blood in the intervillous space because of the same circulatory factors implicated in the pathogenesis of subchorionic fibrin. Hypoxia and acidosis have also been considered in its pathogenesis. Massive perivillous fibrin deposition has been described in some cases of recurrent pregnancy failure.[6] Perivillous fibrin is referred to as "Rohr's fibrinoid" by some authors.[6]

3. *Intravillous fibrinoid* (also called "fibrinoid necrosis of villi"). Intravillous fibrinoid may replace the villi particularly or completely (Figure 18). It normally involves about 3% of the villi in a term placenta. Immunologic factors and degenerative changes in the villi (particularly the cytotrophoblast) have been implicated in its pathogenesis. Antigen–antibody reactions

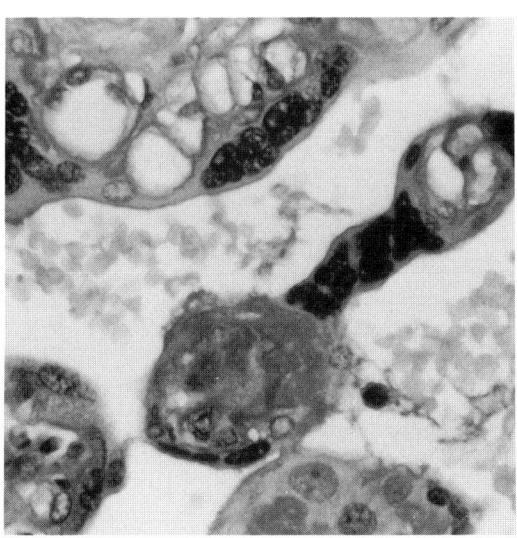

FIGURE 18. Intravillous fibrinoid replacing the villus. Note also the syncytial bridge between the adjacent villi (H&E, ×250).

in the villous stroma have been suggested as the immunologic factors. Burstein et al.[8] have demonstrated stromal binding of insulin in maternal diabetes and anti-D antibodies in Rh isoimmunization.

4. *Fibrinoid deposit in the cell islands and septa.* Degeneration of and secretion by the extravillous trophoblast has been implicated in the pathogenesis of fibrinoid at this location (Figures 9 and 10).
5. *Intervillous fibrin or thrombus.* This appears as a grossly visible 2–5-cm thrombus in the intervillous space. Villi are absent within the focus of the intervillous fibrin (unlike perivillous fibrin) (Figure 19). Nucleated red blood cells (RBCs) can be detected in these thrombi on careful examination (Figure 20). Fox[4] has suggested that fetal bleeding into the intervillous space and its admixture with maternal blood occurring as a result of rupture of the thinned syncytiotrophoblast leads to thrombus formation.
6. *Superficial fibrinoid of the basal plate (Rohr's stria).* This consists of homogeneous or lamellar material in the superficial portion of the basal plate. It forms a discontinuous layer of variable thickness and is probably derived from maternal fibrinogen and degeneration of cells of the basal plate.
7. *Uteroplacental fibrinoid of the basal plate (Nitabuch's stria).* This type of fibrinoid is located in the deeper part of the basal plate at the maternofetal junctional zone, forming a continuous layer up to 100 μm in thickness (Figure 11). Because of its location at the maternofetal (uteroplacental) interface, an immunologic mechanism has been implicated in its pathogenesis.

EXAMINATION OF THE PLACENTA IN THE CLINICAL SETTING

The obstetrician or his/her designee should inspect *all* placentas for gross abnormalities such as incompleteness of the maternal surface, retroplacental hematoma, cord hematoma, rupture of the vasa previa (placental blood vessels coursing over the internal os of the cervix), meconium staining of the amniotic

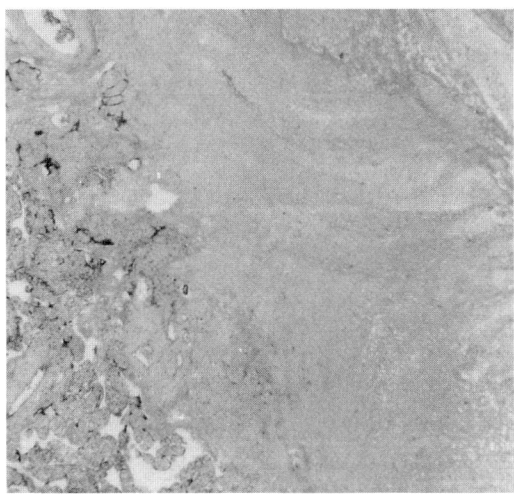

FIGURE 19. Intervillous fibrin (thrombus) (H&E, ×40).

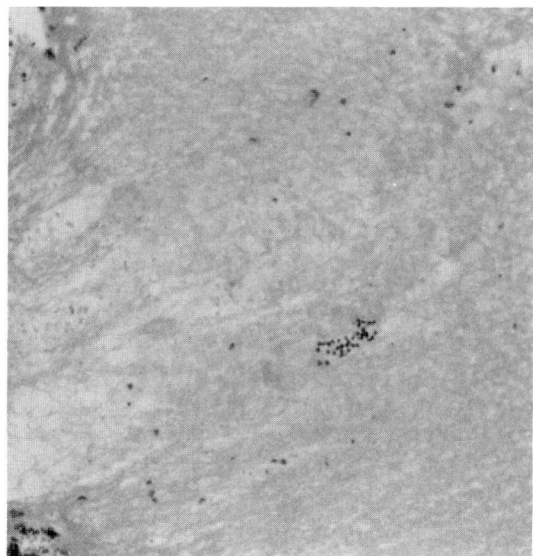

FIGURE 20. Intervillous fibrin (thrombus). Note the cluster of fetal nucleated RBCs (H&E, ×250).

fluid and/or fetus, evidence of intrauterine discharge of meconium by the fetus, etc., and record the findings in the infant's and mother's charts.[9] The umbilical cord length is measured (this is the only occasion when the cord's length can be accurately recorded since a portion of the cord may be retained to collect cord blood). Triaging of, fresh specimen is done as necessary. The samples include chorion, amnion, or fetal skin in the cases of stillbirth for cytogenetics, cultures from the placenta and membranes in cases in which villitis and chorioamnionitis are suspected; and preferably in all cases of premature labor and delivery by taking a swab from the space between amnion and chorion, snap freezing a portion of placental tissue for metabolic disease, etc. The triaging can be done by the pathologist in special cases if the specimen is sent promptly to the pathologist with the information regarding specific requirements of the case.

The placentas from patients with the indications recommended below are sent to the pathologist for further gross and microscopic examination. In some institutions all placentas are sent to the pathologist, who carries out the examination in those cases in which it is requested by the obstetrician. The remaining placentas are stored in the refrigerator at 4°C for 7 days. Those placentas which the clinician subsequently requests a complete pathologic examination can then be retrieved. In some institutions the pathologist decides which of the placentas sent to him/her need a detailed examination.

CLINICAL DATA TO BE SENT TO THE PATHOLOGIST

The following data should be included in the surgical pathology request form: gestational age, pregnancy-related or preexisting maternal disease if any, maternal substance abuse, diagnostic and therapeutic procedures involving the placenta performed during pregnancy, abnormalities related to amniotic fluid, labor and delivery, fetal and/or neonatal abnormalities (low Apgar score, deceleration, growth retardation), and placental abnormalities noted by the obstetrician.[2] If there was placental abruption, it is advisable to indicate on the form the approximate blood loss noted clinically. In abruptio placentae, a blood clot adherent to the maternal surface and producing a depression on it may not always be present.

INDICATIONS FOR PATHOLOGIC EXAMINATION

Placentas are referred to the pathologist for the following reasons:[10] (1) diagnosis of maternal (e.g., preeclampsia, infection) and fetal/neonatal (e.g., Rh immunization, infection) disease, (2) prognosis—prediction of the outcome of the present pregnancy (fetal or neonatal sepsis) and subsequent pregnancies (recurrence of infection), (3) investigation of placental abnormalities in relatively recently recognized maternal diseases with a possible or probable effect on the pregnancy outcome (e.g., lupus anticoagulant, maternal drug abuse, HELLP [hemolysis, elevated liver (enzymes), (low) platelet (count)] syndrome, maternal HIV infection, and (4) legal considerations.

As indicated above, the initial gross inspection and recording of the findings are done by the obstetrician. The indications for pathologic examination can be categorized as follows:[10]

1. *Maternal conditions:* for example, toxemia of pregnancy, diabetes mellitus (or glucose intolerance), hypertension, premature delivery (≤32 weeks' gestation; prematurity is usually defined as gestational age of ≤37 weeks, but for the purpose of placental examination the cutoff point is considered to be 32 weeks by the working group on indications for placental examination of the College of American Pathologists' conference on Placental Examination),[10] prolonged pregnancy (postmaturity: >42 weeks), a history of reproductive failure (abortion, stillbirth), oligohydramnios, prolonged, premature, or preterm rupture of membranes, fever, systemic or localized infection (of the genital tract, etc.), substance abuse, repetitive bleeding, abruptio placentae.
2. *Fetal conditions:* perinatal morbidity and death, stillbirth, multiple births, varnishing twin, congenital anomalies, suspected or known metabolic disorder, growth retardation, meconium staining, immune or nonimmune hydrops fetalis, admission to a neonatal intensive care unit, neurologic problems, suspected or demonstrated infection.
3. *Placental conditions:* for example, any gross abnormality of the placenta, cord or membranes, placenta accreta, or placenta previa.
4. *Miscellaneous:* any case in which there is reason to suspect abnormal pregnancy and a potential for litigation. The placenta shoud be examined in all cases in which invasive procedures such as amniocentesis, percutaneous umbilical blood sampling, or intrauterine fetal transfusion have been performed.

PATHOLOGIC EXAMINATION OF THE PLACENTA

The placenta is examined either in the unfixed or fixed state. Most pathologists prefer the former. The fixed specimen has the merit of having a firmer tissue, which is easier to handle. But the delay entailed by the additional step of fixation makes it impractical for the surgical pathologist. It is, however, essential to fix the placenta from HIV-infected mothers (or from mothers with a history of hepatitis) for at least 3 days. Multiple incisions are made in the placenta from such a patient before immersing it in formalin. A special method of fixation by perfusion for carrying out histomorphometric studies has been described by Jauniaux et al.[11] Benirschke[1] recommends that black-and-white photographs be taken when abnormalities are noted on gross examination. If photography is not feasible, a diagram of the salient abnormal features may be included in the gross examination.

Gross Examination

The following general features are noted:[4] *abnormalities of configuration*—e.g., accessory lobe (smaller than the main placenta), bilobate (virtually equal-sized lobes); (2) *abnormalities of type*—extrachorial (circummarginate, circumvallate) (Figure 21), membranous, etc.; (3) *abnormal cord insertion*—marginal, velamentous, etc.; (4) *umbilical cord*—color, edema, hematoma, trauma, torsion, stricture, true and false knots, length (preferably to be noted by the obstetrician), diameter, number of blood vessels, etc.; (5) *extraplacental membranes*—location of the site of rupture (distance from the placental margin), translucency, meconium staining, amniotic bands, amnion nodosum, exudate, any unusual areas of thickening (? fetus papyraceous), etc.

The next step is to trim the membranes and cord from the placenta and weigh the placenta. Fox[4] expresses reservations about the usefulness of placental weight since it is difficult to assess the weight accurately due to variable amounts of residual maternal and fetal blood in the placenta (maternal: 50–100 g at term; fetal, 25–270 g at term). Fox et al.[12] have shown that formalin fixation of the placenta for 24 hours increases its weight by 7.67%. The weight of the fresh

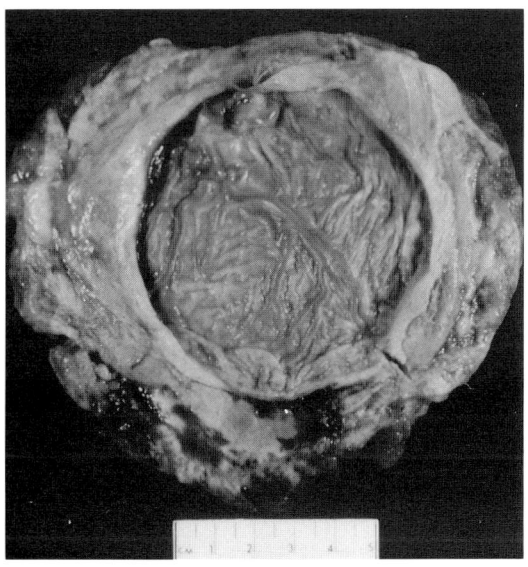

FIGURE 21. Circumvallate placenta. Note that the chorionic plate is smaller than the basal plate, and there is thickening at the site of insertion of the membranes.

placenta can be determined by the following formula: Fresh weight = fixed weight × 0.929.

The next step is to examine the fetal surface of the placenta for the following features: translucency and color of the membranes covering it, amnion nodosum, subamniotic hemorrhage, tuberous projections (indicative of subchorial thrombosis), palpation of large blood vessels for thrombosis, traumatic damage of blood vessels, chorionic septal cysts on the fetal surface, membranous septum and vascular anastomoses in fused twin placentas (see the section on twin placentas for details of the demonstration of anastomosis), and subchorionic fibrin deposition.

The maternal surface is then examined for completeness, tears, calcification, plaques, adherent blood clot, depression, etc. A few thin blood clots are frequently attached to normal placentas. A few small tears are not uncommon in normal placentas. In normal placentas the torn portions can be brought together to demonstrate completeness of the placenta. Thus there are no missing portions. However, in certain conditions, such as placenta accreta, there may be missing portions on the maternal surface.

Serial sections of placenta leaving the tissue attached at the fetal surface made at 0.5–1-cm intervals are examined for septal cysts, intervillous thrombus (round or oval soft, dark lesion), subchorionic fibrin plaques (whitish, firm areas), plaques of perivillous fibrin (firm to hard white, yellowish or brownish white lesion), recent infarct (dark red, firm, roughly triangular lesion) or old infarct (firmer brown to yellow or white lesion), and areas of pallor (corresponding to areas supplied by a thrombosed fetal stem artery). A recent infarct is easier to palpate than to visualize in the unfixed placenta.

Sections for Histologic Examination

The cut surface of the placenta is equally divided into subchorionic/fetal, intermediate, and maternal zones. The villi are best assessed for maturity and other features in the sections taken to include the central part of the maternal zone. The villi close to the maternal surface are the most mature and are involved maximally in gas transfer. Villous density is highest in this area. (See Table 1 and Figures 6 to 8 and 23 to 28 for details of the structure of villi and their proportion in the normal mature placenta.) If an inadequate number of maternal arteries are present in the decidua in the initial sections, additional sections of membrane rolls and maternal surface may be taken in the hope of finding an adequate number of maternal arteries. The various histologic features to be assessed in the section of the placenta are given in Table 2.

The following recommendations for histologic sections are made on the basis of personal experience and those of Altshuler[3] and Fox:[4]

1. Two rolls of membranes are placed in one cassette (each roll is prepared in such a way that the margin of the site of rupture is in the center of the roll). It is essential to include both amnion and chorion in the histologic section. If the membranes are already stripped when the placenta is sent to the pathology laboratory, much of the chorion may be missing. Portions of membranes attached at the margin of the placenta will have both amnion and chorion in such instances. If it is suspected that chorion may be completely stripped from the amnion, several strips from the fetal surface of the placenta (i.e., the

TABLE 1 Types of Villi and Their Structure

Type	Structure	Term placenta
Stem villi	Condensed fibrous stroma, arteries, veins, and branches with media or adventitia (stem villi connect the chorionic plate with the villous tree)	20–25% of villous volume formed by these villi
Mesenchymal villi	Most primitive villi present in the first stages of pregnancy; there is loosely arranged stroma with mesenchymal cells, Hofbauer cells, and poorly developed capillaries	<1% of villous volume formed by these villi
Immature intermediate villi	Bulbous villi, which are a continuation of stem villi; these prevail in immature placentas; they have reticular stroma with numerous channels containing Hofbauer cells, capillaries, and vessels; these villi appear around the 8th week	0–5% of villous volume formed by these villi
Mature intermediate villi	Long, slender villi with blood vessels not having a media or adventitia; occasional stromal channels without macrophages are present	~25% of volume at term formed by these villi
Terminal villi	Final grape-like ramifications of mature intermediate villi; these villi have a high degree of capillarization and are the main site of gas and nutrient exchange	50% of villous volume normally formed by these villi

chorionic plate) should be taken for histologic examination. Assessment of the membrane for chorioamnionitis is incomplete unless chorion is present in the sections. A cross section of the umbilical cord a few centimeters from the insertion should be included in this cassette (Figure 22).

2. Two sections of the central part of the placenta, including the maternal surface, are placed in the second cassette.
3. One section from the central part of the placenta, including the fetal surface, and one cross section from the middle segment of the cord are placed in the third cassette.

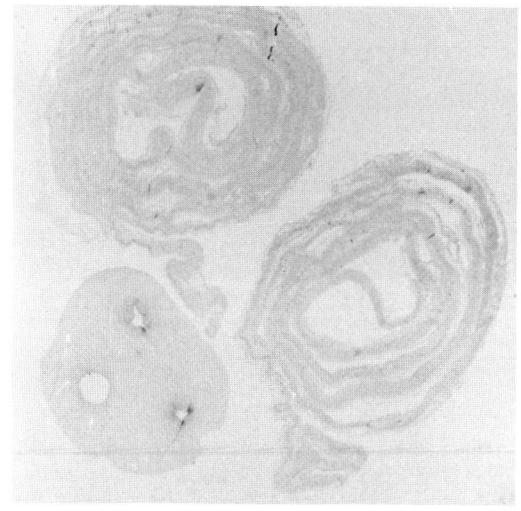

FIGURE 22. Two membrane rolls and a cross section of the umbilical cord are placed in one cassette.

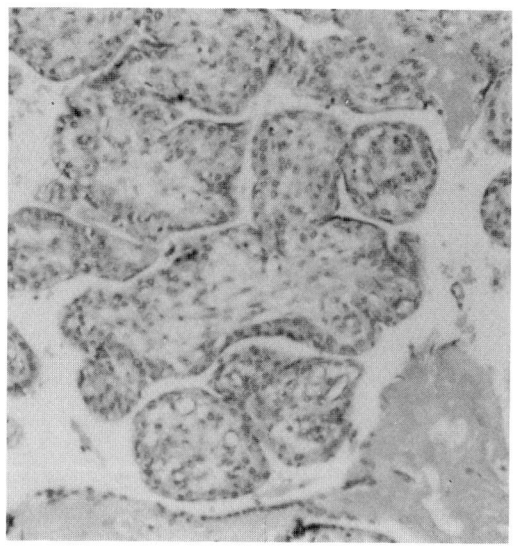

FIGURE 23. Mesenchymal villi composed of loosely arranged stroma with mesenchymal cells and poorly developed capillaries (H&E, ×250).

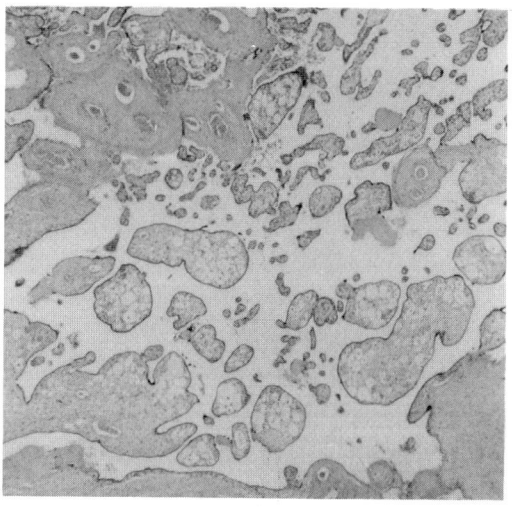

FIGURE 24. Immature intermediate villi with a bulbus outline. Numerous stromal channels containing Hofbauer cells can be seen (H&E, ×40).

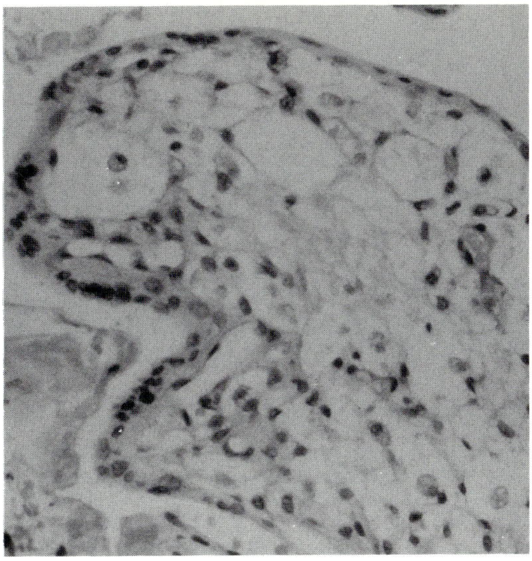

FIGURE 25. Immature intermediate villus showing reticular stroma with numerous channels. Hofbauer cells are present in some of these channels. A few capillaries are seen (H&E, ×250).

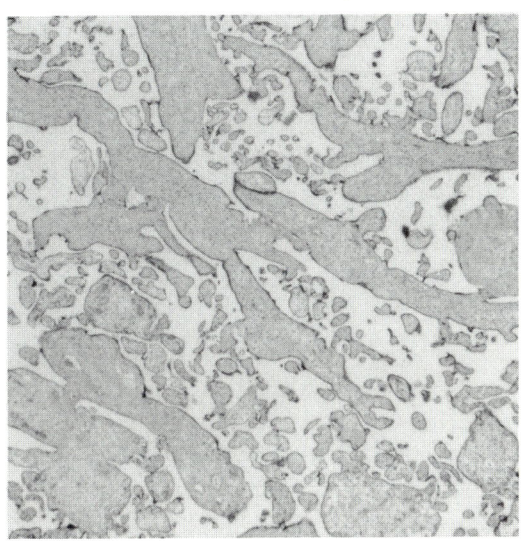

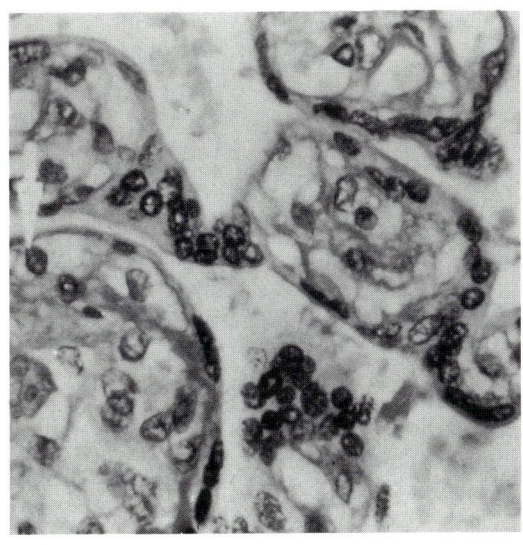

FIGURE 26. Mature intermediate villi with a long, slender shape.

FIGURE 27. Syncytial knots and cytotrophoblastic hyperplasia in a terminal villus. Note also the syncytial bridge and the thickened trophoblastic basement membrane (PAS, ×250).

TABLE 2 Histologic Assessment of the Placenta

Structure	Features to be assessed	Comment
Villi	Maturity, vascularity, nucleated RBCs in capillaries (normally not seen after 30 weeks' gestation), extent of syncytial knots, cytotrophoblastic hyperplasia, trophoblastic basement membrane thickening, deficiency of the vasculosyncytial membrane, stromal fibrosis or edema, Hofbauer cells, intravillous fibrinoid, inflammation, infarction, tumors (hemangioma)	Maturity is best assessed in sections from the central portion of the maternal surface; PAS stain and trichrome stain may be done for assessment of basement membrane and stromal fibrosis; vascularity may be reduced, increased or virtually obliterated
Fetal stem arteries	Thrombosis, obliterative endarteritis, fibromuscular sclerosis, hemorrhagic endovasculitis	These lesions are considered to form a spectrum of fetal vascular obliterative lesions
Chorionic plate	Inflammatory infiltrate in the plate and in the undersurface of the chorionic plate, vasculitis, macrophages containing brown granular pigment (meconium vs. hemosiderin), amnion nodosum, chorionic cyst, remnant of yolk sac, tumors (teratoma, hemangioma)	Iron stain may be done to distinguish between meconium and hemosiderin; in some cases of chorioamnionitis, inflammation may be seen only in the undersurface of the chorionic plate, with or without inflammation of the plate itself
Intervillous space	Perivillous fibrin, intervillous thrombus, inflammatory infiltrate, abnormalities of maternal RBCs (sickling, malarial parasites), collapse, metastatic tumor cells from maternal malignancies (leukemia, melanoma, etc.)	Collapse of the intervillous space in a fairly well-demarcated area is one of the earliest features of placental infarction

TABLE 2 (Continued)

Structure	Features to be assessed	Comment
Basal plate	Excessive fibrin in maternal floor infarction, absence or inadequacy of decidua basalis in placenta accreta, lesions of maternal arteries (thrombi, acute atherosis, arteriosclerosis)	In maternal floor infarction excessive fibrin extends into the intervillous space close to the basal plate; maternal arteries may be present only in the sections of decidua basalis
Membranes	Inflammation, macrophages containing brown granular pigment, amnion nodosum, remnant of yolk sac, maternal arteries in the attached decidua parietalis.	Chorion must be present in the sections for assessment of acute chorioamnionitis; chorion can also be assessed in the sections from the fetal surface; maternal arteries are best seen in the decidua attached to the membranes
Umbilical cord	Number of arteries, vasculitis, funisitis, edema and hemorrhage of Wharton's jelly, absence of Wharton's jelly (in torsion or coarctation of the cord), thrombosis of umbilical blood vessels, vascular tear, macrophages containing brown granular pigment, calcification, necrosis of the muscle coat, embryonic epithelial and vascular remnants, tumors (teratoma, hemangioma)	Vascular changes (thrombosis, tears) should be carefully looked for on the placental side of the knot in the cord and in traumatic lesions; tortuosity and twists in the cord may result in umbilical blood vessels being cut in multiple planes, giving a spurious impression of supernumerary vessels.

4. Separate sections for histologic examination of the decidua cannot be taken since the decidua is attached to the maternal surface of the placenta and to the membranes. It can be assessed histologically in the sections of the membrane rolls and in those taken from the maternal surface of the placenta. Thus three cassettes are routinely taken in every placenta. More sections may be necessary when any of the aforementioned abnormalities are noted on gross examination of the placenta. In a twin placenta, sections of the T zone at the attachment of the septum to the fetal surface and a roll prepared from the septum should be taken. Hematoxylin and eosin stain is used in routine cases. PAS (periodic acid-Schiff) staining to assess thickening of the basement membrane and trichrome staining to assess stromal fibrosis of the villi may be done when indicated.

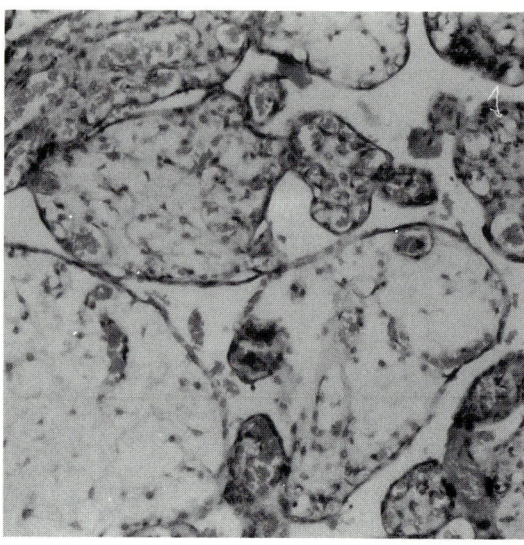

FIGURE 28. Edema of villi. Note the similarity to immature intermediate villi.

Surgical Pathology Report

Attempts should be made to send a report that is complete and concise. To achieve this goal, I have used the format for reporting the results of gross and microscopic examination given in Appendix 1. If a particular gross or microscopic lesion requires further clarification, a comment is added. If a particular lesion which is expected on the basis of the clinical history (e.g., retroplacental hematoma in a case of abruptio placentae) is not found, a negative statement to that effect is included in the gross and/or microscopic description. If a particular gross or histologic finding cannot be adequately assessed (e.g., completeness of the placenta on gross examination or acute atherosis in preeclampsia because of an inadequate number of maternal arteries), this is stated.

Retention of the Specimen

The entire fixed specimen, blocks, slides and reports should be retained according to institutional guidelines.[2] It should be kept in mind that in some states litigation for perinatal cases can be filed for up to 18 years after alleged medical negligence.[13]

GROSS ABNORMALITIES OF THE PLACENTA

Fox[4] divides these into three categories: (1) lesions due to disturbances of maternal blood flow, (2) lesions due to disturbances of fetal blood flow, and (3) noncirculatory lesions (Table 3). It should be noted that many of these lesions can be present in the normal placenta.

Lesions Due to Disturbances of Maternal Blood Flow

Perivillous Fibrin
1. *Gross features.* These lesions represent firm to hard, sharply demarcated, irregularly outlined, yellowish or brownish white plaques, most frequently at

```
                                    SURGICAL PATHOLOGY REPORT
                                        PATHOLOGY #:    IS-93-XXXX
PATIENT:                                       RACE:
MR #:                       ACCT #:
LOCATION:                        DOB:          AGE/SEX:
IMR:463
PRE-OP DIAGNOSIS:
POST-OP DIAGNOSIS:
HISTORY & CLINICAL INFORMATION:

OPERATION PERFORMED:
DATE OF OPERATION:
                                    WERE CULTURES TAKEN?

SPECIMEN SUBMITTED:  1:   PLACENTA

SPECIAL ANATOMIC STUDIES REQUESTED:

ORDERING PHYSICIAN (S):
ATTENDING PHYSICIAN:
COPY TO PHYSICIAN (S):
                                    SURGICAL PATHOLOGY REPORT
                                           DATE DICTATED:
DATE RECEIVED:                             DATE TRANSCRIBED:

GROSS:     Received is one specimen labeled "placenta".
Weight after trimming the membranes and the umbilical cord:
Measurements:
Fetal surface:
Vascular anastomosis:
Maternal surface:
Cut surface:
Membranes:
Cord:       a)  Length -
            b)  Diameter -
            c)  Insertion -
            d)  Number of blood vessels -
            e)  External surface -
            f)  Cut surface -
Loose blood clots:

SUMMARY OF SECTIONS:

MICROSCOPIC:  The following features are noted:  1) Membranes:
         2) Umbilical Cord:     3) Placenta (chorionic plate,
placental blood vessels, villi, intervillous space, placental septa,
cell islands, maternal surface):    4) Maternal arteries in the
decidua (attached to the membranes and/or the basal plate):
```

APPENDIX 1. Format for reporting gross and microscopic findings of the placenta.

the margin of the placenta, measuring up to a few centimeters in their maximum dimension.

2. *Histology.* Fibrin lamellae surrounding viable villi are seen in recent lesions (Figure 16). This is followed by progressive fibrosis and obliteration of blood vessels of the villi (Figure 17). In older lesions the syncytiotrophoblast disappears, but there is cytotrophoblastic proliferation around the circumference of the villi.

3. *Incidence.* It is seen in 22% of full-term placentas and is uncommon in premature placentas. The incidence of *microscopic* perivillous fibrin deposition is virtually 100%, and many of these deposits are visible grossly, according to Benirschke and Kaufmann.[5] There may be massive perivillous fibrin deposition extending to the deeper portions of the placenta in some cases of maternal floor infarction (see below).

TABLE 3 Basic Gross Lesions[a] of the Placenta[4]

Lesions due to disturbances of maternal blood flow to or through the placenta
  Perivillous fibrin
  Subchorionic fibrin
  Massive subchorial thrombosis (Brues' mole)
  Retroplacental hematoma
  Marginal hematoma
  Placental infarct
Lesions due to disturbances of fetal blood flow to the placenta
  Intervillous thrombus
  Kline's hemorrhage
  Fetal artery thrombosis
  Subamniotic hematoma
Noncirculatory lesions
  Calcification
  Chorionic cysts

[a] Many of these "lesions" can be present in the normal placenta or may not be sufficiently extensive to be of clinical signficance.

4. *Pathogenesis.* Fibrin deposition occurs due to eddy currents and stasis within the intervillous space.
5. *Significance.* Since the placenta has a good reserve capacity, loss of ≤30% of the villous population does not have any effect on fetal oxygenation or growth. Therefore, lesions of moderate size are of no clinical significance. Large areas of involvement of the placenta may be associated with fetal loss.[6]

Subchorionic Fibrin

1. *Gross features.* These lesions appear as firm to hard, white, laminated plaque(s) in the subchorionic area. Fresh thrombus may be seen at its border with the placental parenchyma.
2. *Histology.* Laminated fibrin is seen under the chorionic plate. No villi are included in it (Figure 15).
3. *Incidence.* It is seen in ~20% of placentas.
4. *Pathogenesis.* Turbulence, stasis, and eddy currents in the subchorionic zone where there is a change in the direction of maternal blood flow have been implicated as the pathogenetic factors.
5. *Significance.* These lesions are of no clinical significance. Some investigators consider subchorionic fibrin measuring >1 cm in thickness and involving >50% of the placenta as abnormal.

Subchorial Thrombosis (Brues' Mole)

1. *Gross features.* This lesion appears as bulging protuberances on the fetal surface produced by nodular and red thrombus formation in the subchorionic zone. The lesions may be massive, involving a large portion of the subchorionic zone, or may be small in size.
2. *Histology.* The lesion consists of laminated fibrin intermingled with red blood cells (Figure 29). No villi are present within the lesion. The lesion

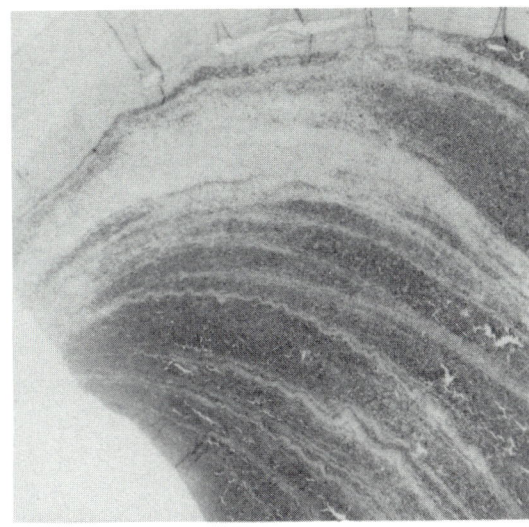

FIGURE 29. Subchorial thrombosis (H&E, ×40).

should be distinguished from subamniotic hematoma, which is between the amnion and the chorion, and histologically there is hemorrhage alone, with no thrombus formation.
3. *Incidence.* It is difficult to assess the true incidence. The lesion in its massive form was first described in placentas of abortuses.
4. *Pathogenesis.* It is suggested that the pathogenesis is related to sudden, marked slowing of blood flow in small or large areas of the subchorionic zone.
5. *Significance.* It may play a role in the abortion. However, Shanklin and Scott[14] demonstrated the presence of massive lesions in placentas from advanced pregnancies and from liveborn infants.

Retroplacental Hematoma (RH)
1. *Gross features.* This lesion may involve variable portions of the maternal surface. The percentage of the surface occupied by the hematoma should be estimated. Many hematomas may be small and are more easily demonstrated in the serial sections of the placenta. The hematoma compresses overlying parenchyma, which may be infarcted (Figure 30). The fresh (recent) hematoma is soft, red, and separable from the maternal surface. Such a hematoma may be detached during delivery or transport of the specimen to the laboratory (Figure 31). The detached clot may not be sent to the laboratory. A crater-like depression on the maternal surface is indicative of the previous hematoma that occupied the depression. Part of or the entire blood clot may have a contour similar to that of the crater on the maternal surface and may fit snugly in it. Older hematoma is brown and firm in consistency. It is adherent to the maternal surface and produces a crater (Figure 32). The very recent RH may not produce a depression on the maternal surface. A large amount of blood clot accompanying the specimen is the only clue to the presence of RH. RH should be distinguished from a simple blood clot on the maternal surface, which is usually thin, can be easily removed, and does not produce a depression on the maternal surface.

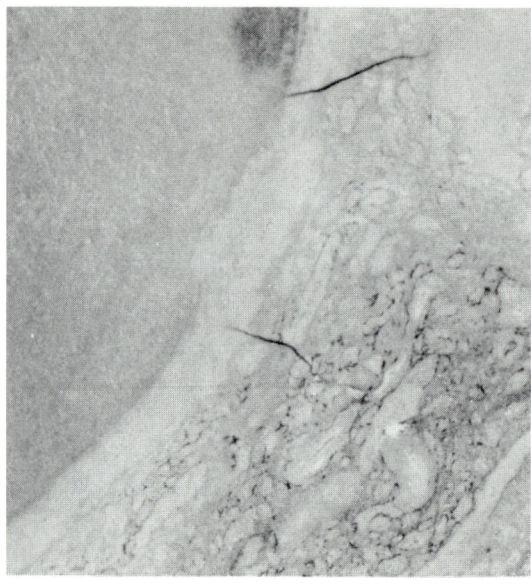

FIGURE 30. Retroplacental hematoma resulting in infarction of the underlying portion of the placenta (H&E, ×40).

2. *Histology.* A blood clot with a few strands of fibrin and a PMN (polymorphonuclear) reaction in the overlying basal plate is seen. In an old hematoma, hemosiderin and macrophages are present. Overlying placental tissue may show infarction (Figure 30).
3. *Incidence.* This lesion is seen in 4.5% of all placentas. The incidence is higher in preeclampsia and in chronic essential hypertension. It is important to note that RH is present in only about 30% of cases of abruptio placentae, and presence of RH is accompanied by the clinical syndrome of abruptio placentae in about 35% of cases.

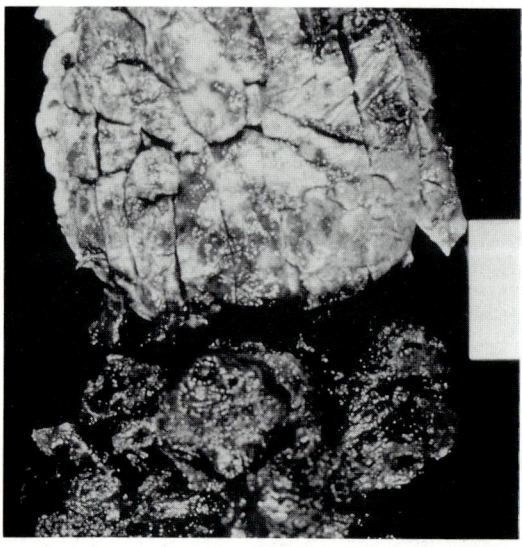

FIGURE 31. Maternal surface of the placenta showing a depression. Note the detached blood clot, which fits well in the depression produced by the retroplacental hematoma.

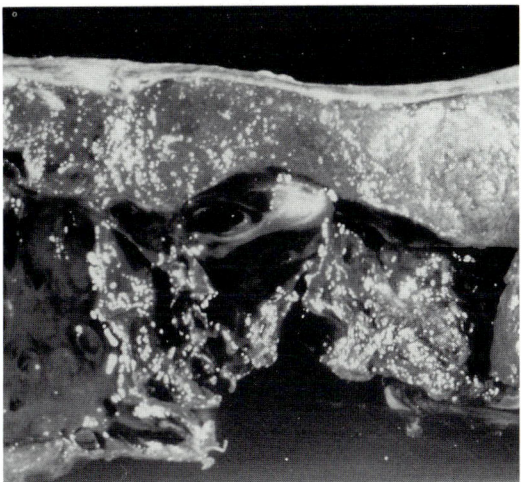

FIGURE 32. Cut section through an older retroplacental hematoma. Note the depression on the maternal surface.

4. *Pathogenesis.* This is not clear. It is generally agreed that RH is due to the rupture of maternal decidual arterioles. It occurs when the arteries are diseased, as in toxemia of pregnancy or hypertension. But it is also seen in cases in which the decidual arteries are normal. It is virtually impossible to demonstrate the ruptured arteriole(s) because of distortion of the decidua. The incidence of abruptio placentae and therefore of RH is increased in maternal cocaine abuse.[15] Obstruction of venous outflow has also been implicated in the pathogenesis of RH. Another theory is that separation of the placenta due to a defective choriodecidual relationship related to folic acid deficiency at the time of conception is the primary event, followed by retroplacental bleeding.

5. *Significance.* A small RH, although it may be accompanied by infarction of the overlying placental parenchyma, is of no significance since there is considerable placental reserve, as noted above. A healthy placenta can withstand a loss of ≤30% of the villous surface. RH involving as much as 30–40% of the maternal surface in an otherwise normal placenta may not adversely affect the fetus. RH in the diseased placenta of toxemia of pregnancy may compromise the placenta further. A hematoma involving 20–25% of the maternal surface of a diseased placenta is considered clinically significant in terms of deprivation of the oxygen supply to the fetus. From the clinical point of view of fetal well-being, loss of the blood supply to the villi due to rupture of the maternal arteriole, and due to their separation from the maternal blood vessels and consequently their infarction, is the most significant aspect of RH. The actual loss of blood is of major concern for the mother's well-being.

It should be noted that RH is a pathologic finding that may or may not be associated with the clinical syndrome of abruptio placentae, which is characterized by abdominal pain and vaginal or concealed bleeding and is usually followed by rapid delivery of the fetus. (In 65% of cases of RH, abruptio placentae does not occur. The converse is also true.) Abruptio placentae may not leave any pathologic imprint on the placenta since most of the blood may find its way around the placental margin and is lost as vaginal bleeding.

Marginal Hematoma
1. *Gross features.* It is seen as a blood clot at the lateral margin of the placenta and may extend to the maternal surface of the membranes and the placenta.
2. *Histology.* Hematoma is seen at the margin of the placenta (Figure 33).
3. *Incidence.* It is seen in 0.74% of all placentas.
4. *Pathogenesis.* It was once considered to be due to rupture of the marginal sinus, which was thought to drain all the blood from the intervillous space into the maternal circulation. It has now been shown that no such marginal sinus exists. Bleeding at the placental margin occurs in placentas that are partially implanted in the inferior segment of the uterus. The hemorrhage results from rupture of uteroplacental veins at the margin, which, as labor progresses, are likely to be torn in the portion of the placenta that is inserted in the lower segment.
5. *Significance.* It is of no clinical significance.

Placental Infarct
1. *Gross features.* A recent infarct is a variably shaped or roughly triangular (base towards the basal plate), well-demarcated, dark red, firm lesion a few millimeters to a few centimeters in size. Infarcts are more commonly seen in the peripheral port. The old infarct is a firmer, brown to yellow or white lesion at 10–14 days of age. A recent infarct is easier to palpate than to visualize in an unfixed placenta. Cystic change may occur in old infarcts.
2. *Histology.* A recent infarct is characterized by a marked reduction in the size of intervillous spaces, with crowding of the villi. The villous capillaries are congested, and there is minimal syncytial necrosis. At a later stage, advanced pyknosis and karyorrhexis of the nuclei of the syncytiotrophoblast are seen and villous capillaries are collapsed. A PMN infiltrate is present around a recent infarct (the PMNs are of maternal origin). With the passage of time, syncytial nuclei disappear. Finally, the syncytiotrophoblast is represented by eosinophilic hyaline material. The villous stroma and capillaries degenerate, but there is no fibrosis. Eventually the old infarct is represented by "ghost" villi. Maternal circulation through the narrowed intervillous space is absent. In the infarct, a small amount of fibrin may be present in the intervillous space. There may be fibrin deposition around the infarct. The arteries in stem villi in the infarct show progressive sclerosis.

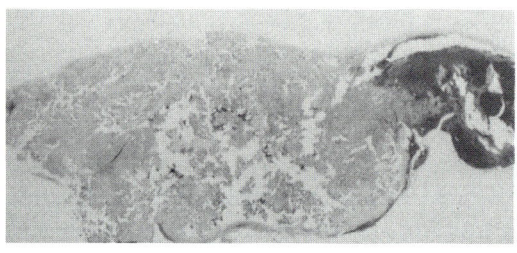

FIGURE 33. Marginal hematoma.

3. *Incidence.* About 25% of normal term placentas contain infarcts involving <5% of the placental parenchyma. The frequency is increased in preeclampsia and hypertension, extensive infarcts being present in 60–70% of patients with severe disease.
4. *Pathogenesis.* The oxygen supply of the villi is derived from the maternal blood (villi develop and grow before they are vascularized by fetal blood vessels, and villi maintain their viability after fetal death). Little or no mixing of blood from individual maternal decidual arterioles occurs. Therefore these arterioles are end arteries. Occlusion of such a blood vessel leads to infarction. Most placental infarcts are due to thrombotic occlusion of the maternal arteries. Infarction also occurs when the blood flow through the placental tissue overlying a retroplacental hematoma is cut off by the latter.
5. *Significance.* The infarcted area in most instances involves <5% of the villous tissue. Only in preeclampsia or hypertension are infarcts involving >5% or more extensive areas seen. With the placental reserve, no compromise of placental function may be seen when as much as 30% of the placental tissue is infarcted if the remaining placenta has a normal blood supply.[16] A diseased placenta, such as in preeclampsia, can withstand the loss of only 15–20% of the villi due to infarction.[4] Extensive placental infarction is associated with a high incidence of fetal hypoxia, intrauterine growth retardation, and fetal death. A centrally localized infarct is of greater significance since the marginal area of the placenta is relatively poorly perfused even normally.

Lesions Due to Disturbance of Fetal Blood Flow

Intervillous Thrombus
1. *Gross features.* Recent thrombus is a round or oval, soft, dark red, 2–5 cm lesion in any part of the placenta. The old thrombus becomes hard and white with lamination. Thrombi of intermediate age have a central soft, cystic-appearing area with a firm, laminated peripheral zone.
2. *Histology.* Recent thrombus contains fibrin lamellae admixed with RBCs. The latter gradually degenerate. Nucleated RBCs are detected in recent thrombi after careful search (Figure 19). Villi are absent within this lesion.
3. *Incidence.* According to different authors, 3–50% of full-term uncomplicated placentas show this lesion.
4. *Pathogenesis.* The thrombi probably consist of an admixture of fetal and maternal blood. It is suggested that fetal bleeding into the intervillous space occurs through the rupture of thinned syncytiotrophoblast covering dilated villous capillaries. Such areas of thinning are found in normal placenta after careful examination. Nucleated RBCs can be demonstrated in the thrombus (Figure 20).[4] Admixture of fetal and maternal blood initiates thrombus formation, especially if the two blood supplies are incompatible.
5. *Significance.* These thrombi have no effect on placental function.

Kline's Hemorrhage
These are hemorrhagic-appearing areas in the placental parenchyma. Nodular foci or foci of semifluid or fluid blood are seen in the lesions. This collection

of blood contains nucleated RBCs. Fox[4] considers the lesion to be a very fresh intervillous thrombus.

Fetal Artery Thrombosis
1. *Gross features.* This lesion is characterized by a triangular area of pallor in the placenta. The thrombosed fetal artery is not demonstrable on gross examination.
2. *Histology.* An area of avascular villi with increased stromal tissue is seen in the histologic section taken from the pale area. Syncytiotrophoblastic knots are prominent. The intervillous space is patent. There is no perivillous fibrin. A thrombosed fetal artery is present in one of the stem villi at the apex of the lesion.
3. *Incidence.* The lesion can be easily overlooked if one is not aware of the existence of such a lesion and if each slice of the sectioned placenta is not examined carefully. It is reported to be present in 4.5% placentas from normal pregnancies. The incidence is about 10% in maternal diabetes.[4]
4. *Pathogenesis.* Thrombosis occurs in an otherwise normal fetal artery. The pathogenesis of thrombosis remains unclear.
5. *Significance.* Single or multiple lesions causing loss of ≤30% villi are of no significance. In rare instances, extensive (40–50%) loss of villi due to multiple fetal arterial thrombi may be the cause of antepartum stillbirth. The thrombi in these cases may show organization.

Subamniotic Hematoma

This appears as a collection of blood between the amnion and chorion on the fetal surface of the placenta. The lesion, which is usually small, is related to trauma of surface veins during delivery arising from possibly excessive traction on the umbilical cord. Most of these hemorrhages are of no clinical significance. However, deSa has described subamniotic hematomas of antepartum origin which were associated with low birth weight.[17] There were old thrombi in the chorionic veins in these cases. Subamniotic hematoma should be distinguished from subchorionic thrombosis. Properly oriented sections of good quality will reveal the precise location (between the amnion and chorion vs. subchorionic) and nature (hemorrhage vs. recent thrombus) of the lesions.

Noncirculatory Lesions

Calcification
1. *Gross features.* These appear as small, firm to hard, scattered, whitish plaques on the maternal surface and give a gritty feel while sectioning if the placenta is heavily calcified.
2. *Histology.* Basophilic material giving a positive reaction on Von Kossa stain for calcium is seen in single villi. Calcification of the trophoblastic basement membrane is seen in placentas of stillbirths and abortions, and occasionally in placentas of normal newborn infants.
3. *Incidence.* Grossly identifiable calcification is seen in 14–37% of placentas at term. The incidence of histologically detectable calcification is higher in

term placentas. It is uncommon before the 36th week of gestation. The incidence of calcification is not higher in postmaturity, preeclampsia, diabetes, and essential hypertension.
4. *Pathogenesis.* There is an association of primigravidity and high maternal serum calcium levels with placental calcification. While dystrophic calcification of dead or degenerative villi occurs, the main form of calcification seen in the placenta is of the metastatic type.
5. *Significance.* There is no known pathologic or clinical significance.

Chorionic Cysts
1. *Gross features.* These appear as 5–10 mm cysts, with gelatinous contents and a membranous wall. Occasionally larger cysts may be present. The cysts are usually seen in the subchorionic zone and the septa. Visible cysts may be present under the fetal surface.
2. *Histology.* The cyst contains structureless eosinophilic material and is lined with an extravillous trophoblast of the septum or the cell islands in which the cyst arises (Figure 34). The chorionic cyst should be distinguished from cystic change in an intervillous thrombus or a chorioangioma.
3. *Incidence.* Chorionic cysts are seen in ~11–20% of placentas. The incidence is higher in edematous placentas and Rh isoimmunization.
4. *Pathogenesis.* The pathogenesis is not clear. It is suggested that colliquative necrosis in the trophoblastic cells and septal tissue leads to cyst formation. Excessive secretory activity of the extravillous trophoblast has also been implicated as a pathogenetic mechanism.
5. *Significance.* The cysts have no clinical significance. They may be visualized on ultrasound if they are sufficiently large.

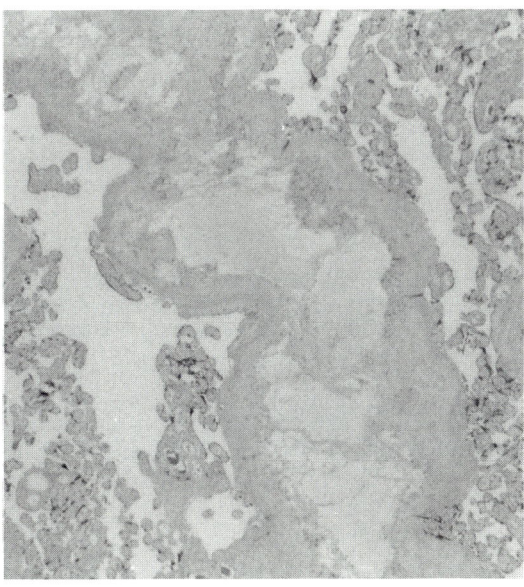

FIGURE 34. Chorionic cyst in a placental septum. Note the faintly staining cystic contents and the extravillous trophoblast lining the cyst (H&E, ×40).

HISTOLOGIC LESIONS OF THE PLACENTA

Fox[4] divides these into lesions of (1) villi, (2) fetal stem arteries, and (3) maternal arteries in the decidua (Table 4). Many of these lesions are present in normal placentas.

Lesions of the Villi Involving Trophoblast

Excessive Number of Syncytiotrophoblastic Knots

1. *Incidence.* The knots are composed of aggregates of small, closely packed, densely staining nuclei protruding from the villous surface into the intervillous space (Figures 8, 27, 35). By electron microscopy the nuclei show degenerative changes. The knots are to be distinguished from syncytial sprouts and syncytial buds.[4] The sprouts are composed of larger collections of syncytiotrophoblast with loosely packed, normally staining nuclei (Figure 35), which probably represent expression of villous sprouting. These sprouts can become detached and enter the maternal circulation. Syncytial buds represent syncytiotrophoblast, which invaginates the underlying stroma. Syncytial bridges are syncytial connections between adjacent villi (Figures 18, 27). It must be emphasized that structures simulating all these types of syncytiotrophoblast can be seen in tangential sections of the villous surface. Syncytial knots are uncommon before 32 weeks' gestation. They increase in number after that period until at term 10–30% of the villi have knots. Knots in >33% of villi are considered excessive. The extent of knots is assessed by counting 100 villi in the histologic section of the placenta taken from the central portion of the maternal zone. The increase in knots with a generalized distribution is seen in postmaturity, preeclampsia, diabetes, hypertension, and antepartum stillbirth. A localized increase is seen in avascular villi secondary to fetal artery thrombosis and in villi adjacent to an infarct. Syncytial knot formation may be normal, reduced or increased in maternal diabetes and Rh isoimmunization.

TABLE 4 Basic Histologic "Lesions"[a] of the Placenta[4]

Lesions of the villi involving
  Trophoblast: excessive number of syncytiotrophoblastic knots, excessive number of cytotrophoblastic cells, deficiency of vasculosyncytial membrane, fibrinoid necrosis of villi
  Trophoblastic basement membrane: thickening of the basement membrane
  Stroma: stromal fibrosis, villous edema, excessive number of Hofbauer cells
  Blood vessels: avascularity, hypovascularity, and hypervascularity (chorangiosis)
  Entire villi: immaturity, accelerated maturation
Lesions of fetal stem arteries
  Fibromuscular sclerosis
  Obliterative endarteritis
  Hemorrhagic endovasculitis
Lesions of maternal arteries of decidua
  Intimal and medial hyperplasia
  Acute atherosis

[a] Many of these "lesions" can be present in the normal placenta.

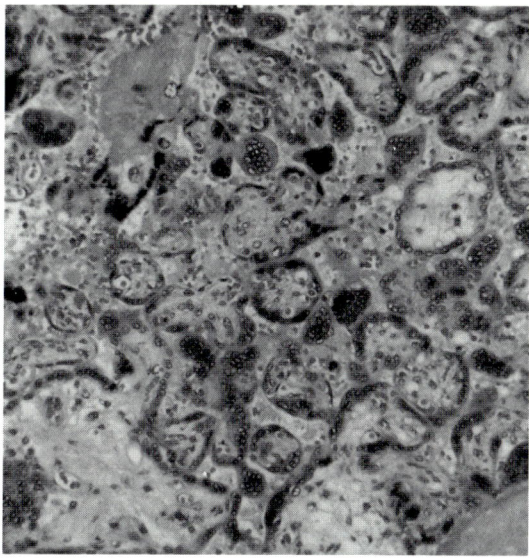

FIGURE 35. Syncytial knots and syncytial sprouts. The former are composed of closely packed, densely staining nuclei and the latter of loosely packed, normally staining nuclei. (H&E, ×100.)

2. *Pathogenesis and significance.* Knot formation is an aging phenomenon. It represents sequestration of aged nuclei. It also occurs as a result of hypoperfusion of villi secondary to obliterative lesions of fetal stem arteries. Hypoperfusion may lead to accelerated aging. Syncytial knots, particularly the bridges they form between adjacent villi, may act as a supportive framework for protection of villous capillaries against sudden changes in intervillous space pressure during labor.

Excessive Number of Cytotrophoblastic Cells
1. *Incidence.* Villous cytotrophoblastic cells that form a complete mantle around immature villi diminish in number with advancing pregnancy. Only a few flattened cytotrophoblastic cells are seen in mature villi. They may be overlooked in the routine H&E-stained slides. Cytotrophoblastic cells are best demonstrated by a PAS stain. Cytoplasm of syncytiotrophoblast IS PAS-positive; that of cytotrophoblast is PAS-negative (Figure 27). The cytotrophoblast is external to the trophoblastic basement membrane. Preparation of thin sections of plastic embedded material also enhances the recognition of cytotrophoblastic hyperplasia. In mature placentas cytotrophoblast is seen in ~20–40% of villi. A greater proportion of villi may show cytotrophoblast in prolonged pregnancy, diabetes, preeclampsia, hypertension, Rh incompatibility and in conditions in which there is fetal hypoxia. It is also seen in low-birth-weight infants and in intrapartum fresh stillbirths after a prolonged period of hypoxia.
2. *Pathogenesis.* It may be due to failure of regression or to proliferation. The latter is present in preeclampsia and hypertension. Cytotrophoblastic hyperplasia appears to be a nonspecific repair phenomenon secondary to damage to syncytiotrophoblast. The syncytial damage is due to placental ischemia, which is present in hypertension and preeclampsia. The extent of cytotrophoblastic hyperplasia is an indicator of the severity of ischemia in these conditions.

Deficiency of Vasculosyncytial Membranes

A distinct thick basement membrane separates the trophoblast from the villous stroma. In some areas the syncytium between knots is thin and without nuclei. In the areas where dilated villous capillaries lie underneath such thin areas, the anuclear thin portion of the syncytium appears to fuse with the vessel wall to form vasculosyncytial membrane (VSM) (Figure 28). These membranes, which are specialized areas of gas transfer, are uncommon until about 32 weeks' gestation. There is a rapid increase in them between 32 weeks and term, when they are present on about 20% of the villi. VSM are not readily demonstrable in areas where the capillaries are collapsed.

1. *Incidence.* Deficiency of VSM is seen in postmaturity, preeclampsia, Rh incompatibility, and diabetes (deficiency is defined as <5% of villi showing VSM).
2. *Pathogenesis and significance.* VSM are a manifestation of villous maturation. In diabetes and Rh incompatibility there is delayed villous maturation. The incidence of fetal hypoxia is higher when VSM are deficient. Deficiency of VSM is also seen in low-birth-weight infants and in stillbirths.

Fibrinoid Necrosis of Villi (Intravillous Fibrinoid)

Homogeneous fibrinoid material is seen beneath the syncytiotrophoblast and external to the basement membrane in the earliest stage of the lesion. An increasing amount of fibrinoid material then appears in the villus, which is finally converted into a fibrinoid nodule with a few attenuated nuclei of syncytiotrophoblast around it (Figure 18). This lesion should be distinguished from perivillous fibrin deposition (Figures 16, 17), in which fibrin is seen around the villi and not within them, as in fibrinoid necrosis of villi.

1. *Incidence.* About 3% of the villi in mature placentas show fibrinoid necrosis. It is more frequently seen in prematurely delivered placentas. It is moderately increased in preeclampsia, diabetes mellitus, and Rh incompatibility. However, excessive intravillous fibrinoid is not seen in essential hypertension.
2. *Pathogenesis.* It may be due to immunologic factors, as indicated above.[8] Degenerative change in the cytotrophoblast as a result of aging of the villi has also been considered as a mechanism.

Lesions of Villi Involving Trophoblastic Basement Membrane

Assessment of thickening (Figure 27) is based on subjective criteria. But on PAS stain one can usually distinguish between normal and thickened basement membrane (Figure 27).

1. *Incidence.* Thickened basement membrane is found in 3% of the villi in about 30% of normal term placentas and in many placentas of prolonged pregnancy. It is seen in a higher proportion of villi in preeclampsia, essential hypertension, diabetes mellitus and Rh incompatibility.
2. *Significance.* It may lead to fetal hypoxia. A higher proportion of villi in the placentas of low-birth-weight infants and intrapartum stillbirths show trophoblastic basement membrane thickening.

3. *Pathogenesis.* It appears to be the result of uteroplacental ischemia, which causes cytotrophoblastic hyperplasia. Excessive basement membrane production accompanies hyperplasia.

Lesions of Villi Involving Stroma

Stromal Fibrosis

1. *Incidence.* There is little collagen in the stroma of mature villi (Figure 8), although ≤3% of villi may be fibrotic in term placentas. In prolonged pregnancy up to 33% of the villi show stromal fibrosis. Stromal fibrosis may be seen in preeclampsia and diabetes mellitus but not in Rh incompatibility.
2. *Pathogenesis.* It is due to reduced blood flow through the villi (it is seen in the villi supplied by an occluded fetal stem artery).
3. *Significance.* There is no association between stromal fibrosis and fetal hypoxia. Stromal fibrosis seen in the placentas of antepartum stillbirths is a secondary change related to cessation of fetal circulation (Figure 36). It is not seen in intrapartum stillbirths.

Villous Edema. Villous edema is characterized by villous swelling and microcystic change in the villous stroma (Figure 28). It appears to be due to distention of stromal channels in the immature intermediate villi.[18] Hofbauer cells are found in these distended channels. Villous edema is a poorly understood entity. Naeye et al.[19] found a high incidence between 25 and 32 weeks of gestation. In their series they reported a good correlation with intrauterine hypoxia. Shen-Schwarz et al.[18] found a significant association of villous edema in term placentas with fetal and neonatal death. In the term placenta, the edema involves the immature intermediate villi, which are present in a small proportion (Table 1). It should be noted that villous edema is also seen in diabetes mellitus. Rh incompatibility, preeclampsia, and placental infections (syphilis, toxoplasmosis, cytomegalovirus (CMV), etc.). The cause of villous edema is

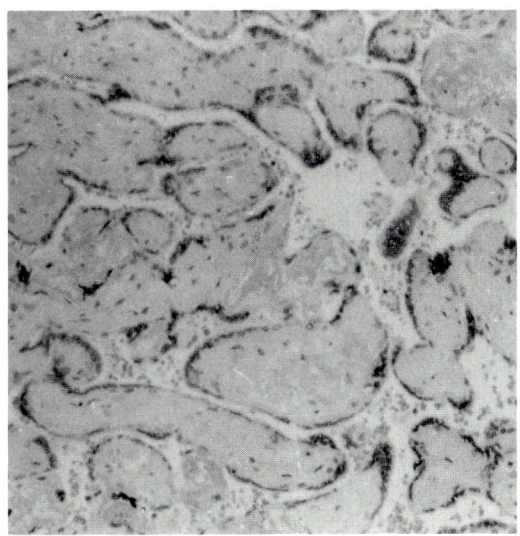

FIGURE 36. Stromal fibrosis of the villi in the placenta of an antepartum, macerated stillborn infant delivered over 2 weeks after fetal death. Note also the avascularity of the villi (H&E, ×100).

diabetes mellitus, Rh incompatibility, and in pregnant women who smoke heavily. It is probably related to hemodynamic changes occurring in the fetal circulation secondary to uteroplacental ischemia. This lesion leads to further reduction in fetal perfusion of the villi, which results in stromal fibrosis.

Hemorrhagic Endovasculitis (HEV)

HEV involves fetal stem arteries, their branches and even villous capillaries. The arteries show medial and intimal hyperplasia with luminal narrowing. Recent or old thrombi may be present. Intact and fragmented RBCs are seen within the vessel wall (Figure 38). HEV is considered a lesion belonging to the spectrum of fetal vascular obliteration. The lesion may be focal or diffuse.[22] An association with stillbirth and intrauterine growth retardation has been found.[23] However, other investigators[24] have not confirmed such an association. The pathogenesis of HEV is not known. Originally viral etiology was implicated.[22,23] Disseminated intravascular coagulation, hypoxia, and poor perfusion have also been suggested as pathogenetic factors. An HEV-like lesion has been observed in placental organ culture. Low oxygen tension at the central core of the villi in the organ culture was considered the pathogenetic mechanism.[25]

Histopathology of Maternal Uteroplacental Arteries

In the early stages of pregnancy, actively proliferating cytotrophoblastic cells infiltrate the decidual portion of the spiral arteries, leading to destruction of elastic and muscle tissue and fibrinoid change in the media. Between 14 and 20 weeks' gestation, cytotrophoblastic infiltration and associated changes in the media extend to the myometrial portion of the arteries. The infiltrated decidual and myometrial portions of spiral arteries become dilated because of destruction of the media (Figure 39). These physiologic changes in the spiral arteries, which augment the blood flow required for progression of the pregnancy, are confined to the placental bed and are not seen in the arteries of the decidua capsularis or decidua parietalis or in the basal arteries. The lesion of "acute atherosis" of

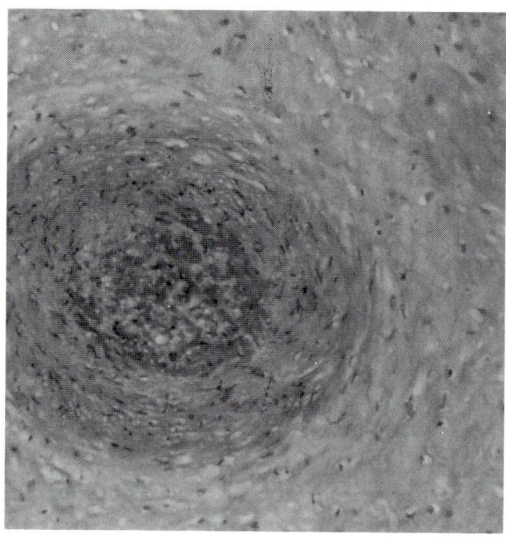

FIGURE 38. HEV characterized by medial and intimal hyperplasia, with RBCs within the vessel wall (H&E, ×40).

3. *Pathogenesis.* It appears to be the result of uteroplacental ischemia, which causes cytotrophoblastic hyperplasia. Excessive basement membrane production accompanies hyperplasia.

Lesions of Villi Involving Stroma

Stromal Fibrosis
1. *Incidence.* There is little collagen in the stroma of mature villi (Figure 8), although ≤3% of villi may be fibrotic in term placentas. In prolonged pregnancy up to 33% of the villi show stromal fibrosis. Stromal fibrosis may be seen in preeclampsia and diabetes mellitus but not in Rh incompatibility.
2. *Pathogenesis.* It is due to reduced blood flow through the villi (it is seen in the villi supplied by an occluded fetal stem artery).
3. *Significance.* There is no association between stromal fibrosis and fetal hypoxia. Stromal fibrosis seen in the placentas of antepartum stillbirths is a secondary change related to cessation of fetal circulation (Figure 36). It is not seen in intrapartum stillbirths.

Villous Edema. Villous edema is characterized by villous swelling and microcystic change in the villous stroma (Figure 28). It appears to be due to distention of stromal channels in the immature intermediate villi.[18] Hofbauer cells are found in these distended channels. Villous edema is a poorly understood entity. Naeye et al.[19] found a high incidence between 25 and 32 weeks of gestation. In their series they reported a good correlation with intrauterine hypoxia. Shen-Schwarz et al.[18] found a significant association of villous edema in term placentas with fetal and neonatal death. In the term placenta, the edema involves the immature intermediate villi, which are present in a small proportion (Table 1). It should be noted that villous edema is also seen in diabetes mellitus. Rh incompatibility, preeclampsia, and placental infections (syphilis, toxoplasmosis, cytomegalovirus (CMV), etc.). The cause of villous edema is

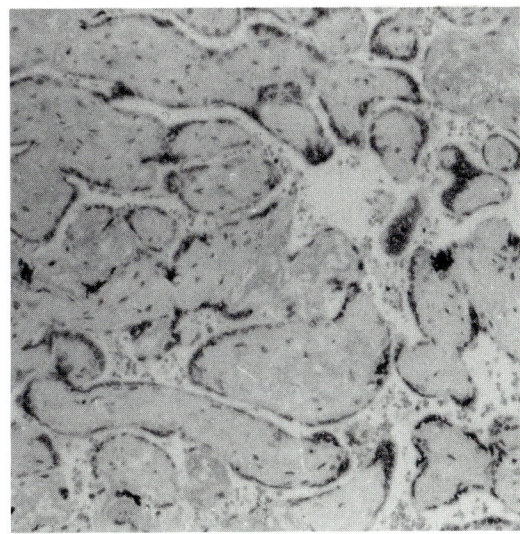

FIGURE 36. Stromal fibrosis of the villi in the placenta of an antepartum, macerated stillborn infant delivered over 2 weeks after fetal death. Note also the avascularity of the villi (H&E, ×100).

unknown. It may be due to functional insufficiency of the fetal circulation. It has been suggested that villous edema may compress the villous capillaries resulting in fetal hypoxia due to decreased fetoplacental blood flow.[19] However, the clinical significance of villous edema remains unclear.

Excessive Number of Hofbauer Cells. Hofbauer cells are tissue macrophages derived from both the mesenchyme of the villi and the circulating blood monocytes. These cells, which are located in stromal channels of the villi (Figure 25), are reduced in number with advancing gestation. However, they can be seen in immature or edematous villi in most term placentas (80%). Hofbauer cells are not seen in fully mature, nonedematous villi. The cells are increased in number in diabetes and Rh incompatibility. Their presence is indicative of villous immaturity or edema.

Abnormalities of Villous Blood Vessels

Avascular villi are present distal to fetal artery thrombosis or as a consequence of intrauterine fetal death (Figure 36). "Villous hypovascularity" implies small, nondilated blood vessels, not in reduction in the number of blood vessels. It is seen in delayed maturation or is secondary to fetal artery thrombosis. Villous hypervascularity occurs in diabetes mellitus, preeclampsia, and Rh incompatibility. Normal villi contain about five vascular channels. Hypervascularity implies an increased number of vascular channels, not mere congestion or dilatation. Altshuler[20] defined quantitative criteria for hypervascularity that he labeled chorangiosis. Chorangiosis is diagnosed when villi, each with 10 or more vascular channels, are seen in ≥10 low-power fields of viable placental tissue in three different placental areas.[20] Chorangiosis is associated with a higher incidence of neonatal morbidity and death and with congenital malformations.

Generalized Abnormalities of Villi

Villous Immaturity. Assessment of villous immaturity is difficult in placentas of <37 weeks' gestation. At term the villi are small and have dilated vessels that compress the stroma. Term villi also show syncytial knots (Figure 8). Immature villi are larger and have small, undilated vessels, a relatively large amount of stroma and no syncytial knots (Figures 24, 25). Immature villi may be present in small, isolated groups among mature villi in a term placenta. This type of distribution is seen in 97% of term placentas and is within normal limits. These immature villi represent newly formed villi, indicating that villous growth continues until term. In the second type of distribution, most of the villi are markedly immature for the gestational age. Delay in maturation occurs in diabetes mellitus, Rh incompatibility, syphilis, and Down's syndrome. The cause of villous immaturity is unknown. The structure of various types of villi and the proportion in which these are normally present in a mature placenta are given in Table 1 and Figures 6–8 and 22–26. Kaufmann et al.[21] have described a number of cases of imminent fetal asphyxia in which there was deficiency of terminal villi in term placentas. A preponderance of long, slender, mature intermediate villi with a paucity of terminal villi was demonstrated by scanning electron and light microscopy.

Accelerated Maturation. This is seen in preeclampsia. It is suggested that it is a compensatory mechanism to counter the effects of inadequate uteroplacental blood flow. Accelerated maturation is also seen in some placentas from premature infants (fetoplacental asynchrony).

The various types of histopathologic lesions involving the villi described above can be divided into three categories based on their pathogenesis: (1) lesions due to reduced uteroplacental blood flow (e.g., in preeclampsia or hypertension)—cytotrophoblastic hyperplasia and trophoblastic basement membrane thickening, (2) lesions due to reduced fetal blood flow—increased syncytial knots and stromal fibrosis, and (3) lesions due to undetermined pathogenesis—fibrinoid necrosis of villi, abnormalities of villous maturation, and lack of VSM.

Lesions Involving Fetal Stem Arteries

Fibromuscular Sclerosis

Marked hyperplasia of fibrous tissue in the intima and of muscle in the media obliterates the lumen (Figure 37). These changes may be localized or generalized. The localized variety is seen in an artery supplying an area of infarct or supplying villi which are embedded in fibrin or in an artery that is distal to an occlusive thrombus. Generalized lesion is seen in the placentas of antepartum stillbirths of long duration. This lesion is a reactive phenomenon secondary to lack of blood flow after intrauterine death.

Obliterative Endarteritis

Intimal hyperplasia in the stem arteries leads to narrowing or almost complete obliteration of the lumen (Figure 37). It is not an inflammatory lesion. This lesion is focally present in 10% of term normal placentas. But it is more commonly and more extensively seen in preeclampsia, essential hypertension,

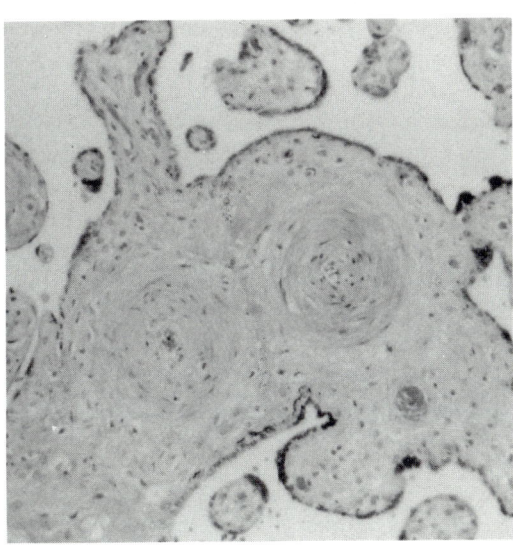

FIGURE 37. Fibromuscular hyperplasia (artery on the right) and obliterative endarteritis (artery on the left) of fetal stem arteries (H&E, ×100).

diabetes mellitus, Rh incompatibility, and in pregnant women who smoke heavily. It is probably related to hemodynamic changes occurring in the fetal circulation secondary to uteroplacental ischemia. This lesion leads to further reduction in fetal perfusion of the villi, which results in stromal fibrosis.

Hemorrhagic Endovasculitis (HEV)

HEV involves fetal stem arteries, their branches and even villous capillaries. The arteries show medial and intimal hyperplasia with luminal narrowing. Recent or old thrombi may be present. Intact and fragmented RBCs are seen within the vessel wall (Figure 38). HEV is considered a lesion belonging to the spectrum of fetal vascular obliteration. The lesion may be focal or diffuse.[22] An association with stillbirth and intrauterine growth retardation has been found.[23] However, other investigators[24] have not confirmed such an association. The pathogenesis of HEV is not known. Originally viral etiology was implicated.[22,23] Disseminated intravascular coagulation, hypoxia, and poor perfusion have also been suggested as pathogenetic factors. An HEV-like lesion has been observed in placental organ culture. Low oxygen tension at the central core of the villi in the organ culture was considered the pathogenetic mechanism.[25]

Histopathology of Maternal Uteroplacental Arteries

In the early stages of pregnancy, actively proliferating cytotrophoblastic cells infiltrate the decidual portion of the spiral arteries, leading to destruction of elastic and muscle tissue and fibrinoid change in the media. Between 14 and 20 weeks' gestation, cytotrophoblastic infiltration and associated changes in the media extend to the myometrial portion of the arteries. The infiltrated decidual and myometrial portions of spiral arteries become dilated because of destruction of the media (Figure 39). These physiologic changes in the spiral arteries, which augment the blood flow required for progression of the pregnancy, are confined to the placental bed and are not seen in the arteries of the decidua capsularis or decidua parietalis or in the basal arteries. The lesion of "acute atherosis" of

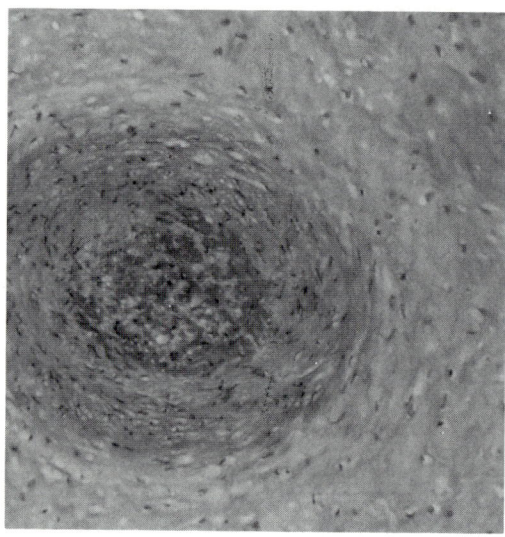

FIGURE 38. HEV characterized by medial and intimal hyperplasia, with RBCs within the vessel wall (H&E, ×40).

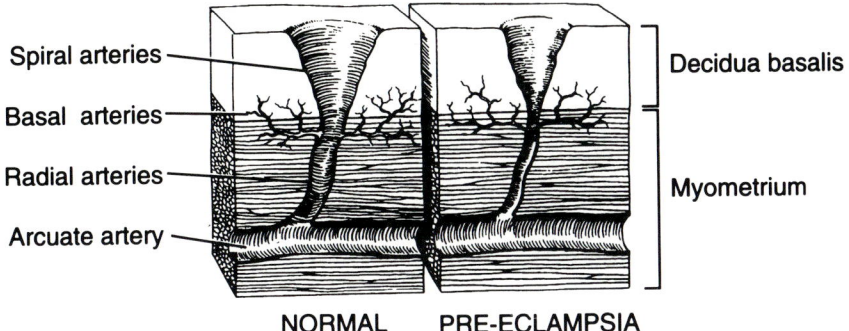

FIGURE 39. Diagrammatic representation of vascular changes in the spiral arteries. Note the dilatation of the artery extending into the myometrium in normal pregnancy. In preeclampsia the arterial dilatation does not extend to the myometrium. (Adapted from Fox H: *Pathology of the Placenta.* Saunders, Philadelphia, 1978, Chap. 6.)

preeclampsia is seen only in the intramyometrial segments of the spiral arteries of the placental bed, in the spiral arteries of the decidua parietalis, and in basal arteries. The intradecidual portions of the spiral arteries of the placental bed are not involved. Thus acute atherosis occurs only in arteries that have *not* undergone the physiologic changes of pregnancy. It is characterized by fibrinoid necrosis and lipophages in the vessel wall with a perivascular lymphomononuclear infiltrate. Thrombosis may also be present (Figures 40, 41). In the initial stages lipid accumulation in the muscle cells of the media is seen on ultrastructural examination. Subsequent necrosis of these cells is followed by release of lipid that is phagocytosed by macrophages.[26,27] The term "acute atherosis" was introduced by Zeek and Assali.[28]

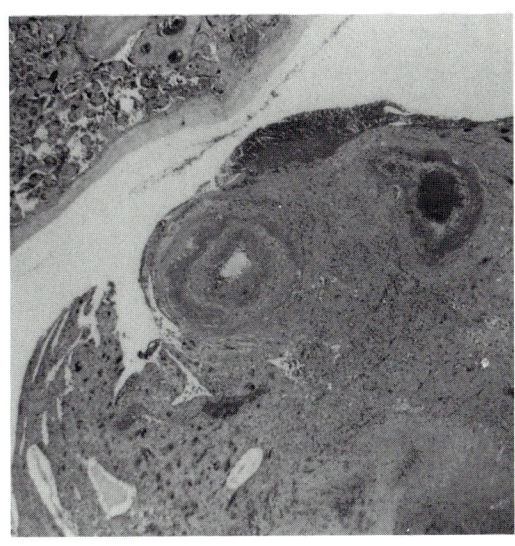

FIGURE 40. Acute atherosis of preeclampsia. Note the fibrinoid necrosis of the spiral arteries (arrow) in the decidua parietalis (H&E, ×5).

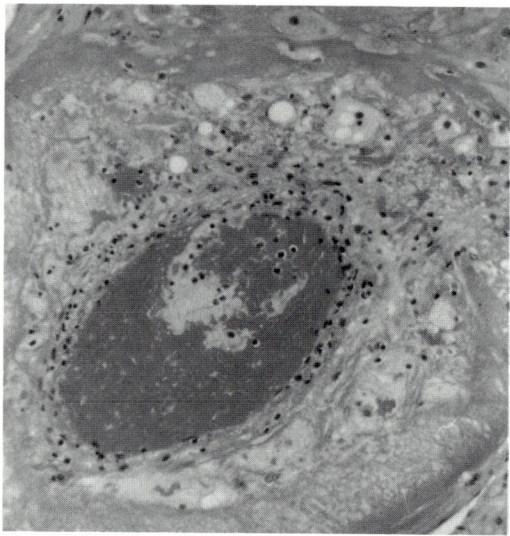

FIGURE 41. Fibrinoid necrosis, foamy macrophages, scattered lymphomononuclear infiltrate, and thrombosis of a basal artery in the decidua basalis (H&E, ×250).

In women with essential hypertension, the maternal arteries in the decidua show thickening of, muscle coat with intimal hyperplasia and narrowing of the lumen (Figure 42). The basal arteries, spiral arteries in the decidua parietalis, and myometrial segments of the spiral arteries of the placental bed are affected by these changes. The intradecidual portions of the spiral arteries of the placental bed do not show these alterations since these arteries have already undergone the changes associated with implantation and placental development described above. If preeclampsia occurs in a patient with preexisting

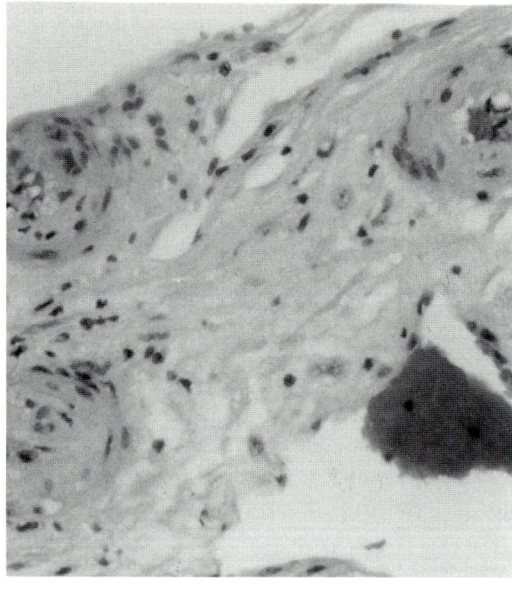

FIGURE 42. Thickening of the muscle coat of the spiral arteries in the decidua parietalis in maternal hypertension (H&E, ×100).

hypertension, acute atherosis is superimposed on the arteriosclerotic changes described above.

As noted above, the blood vessels showing the lesions associated with hypertension and preeclampsia are present in the decidua basalis attached to the maternal surface and to the decidua parietalis attached to the membranes. With enlargement of the embryo, the decidua capsularis merges with the decidua parietalis. The uterine cavity is thus obliterated. The decidua capsularis degenerates and disappears by about 22 weeks of gestation. It is important to assess the decidua attached to the membrane in the membrane rolls prepared for histologic examination and the decidua along the maternal surface for changes in the maternal arteries.

The extent to which each of the gross and histologic abnormalities described above can be seen in the normal term placenta is stated in Table 5.

LESIONS OF THE PLACENTA AS A WHOLE OR OF THE PLACENTAL DISK

Large Placenta

Because of the inconstant amount of blood present in the placenta, placental weight cannot be used as an accurate marker for the large or small placenta.

TABLE 5 Normal Range of Gross and Microscopic Lesions of the Term Placenta

Feature	Normal range
Subchorionic fibrin	Present in 20% of term placentas
Intervillous fibrin (thrombus)	Present in 36% of term placentas
Infarct(s)	Present in 25% of term placentas (involving <5% of the area)
Grossly demonstrable perivillous fibrin	Present in 22% of term placentas (histologically demonstrable perivillous fibrin present in virtually all placentas)
Stromal fibrosis	Seen in ~3% of villi at term
Syncytial knots	Seen in 11–30% of villi at term
Vasculosyncytial membranes (VSM)[a]	Uncommon until 32 weeks; increase rapidly after 32 weeks; at term 20% villi show VSM
Thickened trophoblastic basement membrane	Seen in ~3% of villi in 30% of term placentas
Intravillous fibrin (fibrinoid necrosis of villi)	Seen in ~3% of villi of term placentas
Cytotrophoblast[b]	20% villi at term show inconspicuous, flattened cells.
Fetal artery thrombosis	Seen in 4.5% of term placentas
Obliterative endarteritis	Seen in 10% of term placentas

[a]VSM deficiency: VSM in <5% villi.
[b]Cytotrophoblastic hyperplasia: prominent cytotrophoblast in >20% of villi at term.

However, in practice, the guidelines mentioned below for the diagnosis of large and small placentas may be used. A term placenta weighing >750 g is considered large. The cutoff points for large placentas at other gestational ages are not specified. In general, the diagnosis of large placenta at earlier gestation may be made when the weight of the placenta exceeds the upper limit of normal for the gestational age by 100 g. The normal ranges of weights and means are given in Table 6.[29] This guideline is suggested after taking into consideration the increased weight of the placenta that may be related to the maternal and fetal blood present in it. Large placentas also tend to be pale and large. On histologic examination, the villi are large and appear immature. Villous edema is present. Hofbauer cells are prominent. Large placentas are seen in Rh incompatibility, chronic intrauterine infections, and maternal diabetes.

Small Placenta

The diagnosis of small placenta is made when the weight of the placenta is less than the lower limit of normal for the gestational age (Table 6). A small placenta may have an otherwise normal gross and microscopic appearance, or it may be related to the presence of multiple old infarcts. Small placentas are seen in toxemia of pregnancy, hypertension, multiple congenital anomalies associated with trisomy syndromes, etc. The placenta also tends to be small when there is intrauterine growth retardation.

Extrachorial Placentas

In extrachorial placentas the chorionic plate is smaller than the basal plate. The membranes arise at some distance from the circumference of the fetal surface, leaving a ridge of naked placental tissue projecting beyond the limits of the chorionic plate. There are two types of extrachorial placentas: circummarginate and circumvallate. If the membranes arise without any thickening, the placenta is categorized as circummarginate. If the membranes show a rolled edge

TABLE 6 Weights of Placenta at Various Gestational Ages

	Placental weight (g)	
Gestational (weeks)	Mean ± SD[a]	Range (mean ± 2 S.D.)
28	270 ± 39	192–348
29–30	287 ± 36	215–359
31–32	335 ± 45	245–425
33–34	370 ± 60	253–493
35–36	414 ± 64	286–542
37–38	452 ± 58	336–568
39–40	481 ± 68	345–617
41–42	494 ± 74	346–642
43+	490 ± 62	366–614

[a] S.D. = standard deviation.
Adapted from Reed GB, Clairaux AE, Bain, AD: Diseases of fetus and newborn: *Pathology, radiology and genetics*. Mosby, St. Louis, 1989, p. 207

having a rim of fibrinous material, it is categorized as circumvallate (Figure 21). In some cases the placenta may be marginate in one area and vallate in another. Normal areas may also be seen in these placentas. Histologic examination of the tissue at the membranous attachment in circummarginate placenta shows amnion, chorion and a small amount of fibrin. The fold at the membranous attachment in circumvallate placenta contains amnion, chorion, fibrin, hemorrhage, decidua, and senescent villi. Circummarginate and partially circumvallate placentas are of no particular clinical significance. Total circumvallate placenta is associated with a higher incidence of antepartum bleeding, premature labor, perinatal mortality, and low birth weight. This suggests that the circumvallate placenta is relatively inefficient. The pathogenesis of extrachorial placentation is not clear. The following theories have been suggested: unusually shallow or deep implantation of the ovum, lack of coordination between placental and uterine growth, and hemorrhage around the placental edge.

Placenta Membranacea

In this type, the placenta envelops the entire or greater part of the gestational sac. Thus the membranes are covered on their outer aspect by villi. This type of placenta is extremely rare. It causes recurrent antepartum bleeding with poor fetal survival. The condition results from failure of villous atrophy around the membranes in the early weeks of gestation (see section on development of the placenta above).

Bilobate Placenta

This type of placenta has two approximately equal-sized lobes. The umbilical cord is inserted between the two lobes into the connecting portion of chorionic tissue or velamentously. Bleeding and adherent placenta can occur in this type of abnormality, which is noted in ~2.2% of placentas. Multilobate placenta (three or more lobes) is extremely rare.

Accessory or Succenturiate Lobe

One or more accessory lobes in addition to the main placenta may be present. The accessory lobe may be connected by chorionic tissue or by membranes. The umbilical cord is usually inserted in the main placenta. The incidence of accessory lobes is ~3%. In most cases there is no clinical significance. However, in rare instances (1) the accessory lobe may be retained in the uterus after delivery of the main placenta, causing postpartum bleeding, (2) the accessory lobe may be located over the internal os, causing placenta previa, or (3) it may cause fetal hemorrhage due to trauma to vessels coursing through the membranes to supply the accessory lobe.

Placenta Previa

The placenta is implanted in the lower uterine segment. The placenta precedes the fetus at delivery since it covers the cervical os. It is a clinical disorder. The pathologist cannot make a diagnosis of the site of implantation. Painless uterine bleeding due to mechanical separation of the placenta following retraction of the uterine wall during labor is the principal manifestation. The extent to which the placenta covers the internal os is graded as partial or complete. Rarely, placenta previa accreta may be present.

Placenta Accreta

This is defined as "abnormal adherence, either in whole or part, of the afterbirth to the underlying uterine wall."[30] Placenta accreta may be partial or total, involving the entire maternal surface. Three gradations are recognized: (1) placenta accreta vera, in which the villi are attached to but do not penetrate into the myometrium; (2) placenta increta, in which the villi invade superficial portions of the myometrium (Figure 43); and (3) placenta percreta, in which the villi invade the entire thickness of the myometrium. The characteristic pathologic feature in all categories of placenta accreta is the absence or the marked attenuation of the decidua basalis (Figure 44). Only small groups of decidual cells are scattered in loose connective tissue. The fibinoid layer in the decidua is also attenuated or absent. The attenuation or absence of decidua basalis may be focal. The decidua parietalis may also show the same abnormality.

The clinical features associated with placenta accreta are incomplete or total lack of placental separation and continued bleeding. Manual removal can be successful in many cases, but hysterectomy may occasionally be needed (Figure 44). The maternal surface is often distorted and fragmented in the manually separated placenta accreta. It is difficult to get well-oriented sections in these specimens. However, an attempt should be made to get as well-oriented sections as possible (Figure 43). These sections should be compared with similar sections from a normal placenta (Figures 9, 11) to appreciate the decidual abnormality. The villi are normal and do not show any trophoblastic hyperplasia. The pathologic diagnosis of placenta increta and percreta is made by demonstration of incomplete or complete penetration of the myometrium by

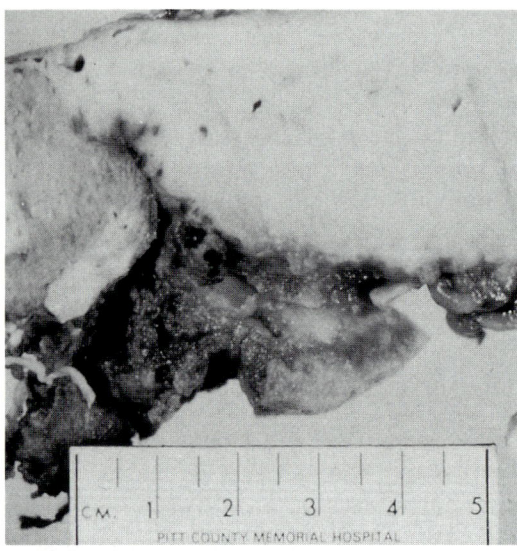

FIGURE 43. Hysterectomy specimen showing placenta increta in which the placental villi invaded the muscle.

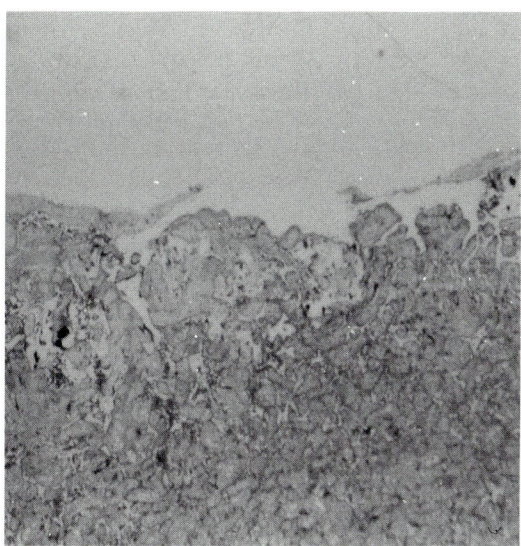

FIGURE 44. Deficient, attenuated decidua basalis in placenta accreta (H&E, ×40).

placental villi. Therefore, pathologic diagnosis of placenta increta and percreta can be made only on a hysterectomy specimen unless a portion of the myometrium is present along the maternal surface of the manually removed, adherent portion of the placenta.

The pathogenesis is related to absence or deficiency of decidual transformation of the endometrium, culminating in the trophoblastic invasion of the placental bed beyond the normal depth. Thus the primary abnormality involves the decidua. The predisposing factors for placenta accreta include (1) a previous history of (a) uterine curettage, (b) cesarean section, (c) manual removal of placenta, (d) uterine sepsis, and (e) uterine surgery; (2) abnormal location of implantation—placenta previa, cornual implantation; and (3) uterine leiomyomas and malformations. In these circumstances, there may be localized deficiency or scarring of endometrium leading to the decidual abnormality during pregnancy. Excessive invasiveness of the villi does not appear to be a factor in the pathogenesis.

Retroplacental Hematoma (RH) and Abruptio Placentae (AP)

These have already been described in the section on gross abnormalities of the placenta. It is important to bear in mind the distinction between RH and AP. The former is a pathologic lesion, the latter a clinical syndrome. Although the former is the pathologic hallmark of the latter, each can be present without the demonstrable presence of the other.

Maternal Floor Infarction

1. *Definition.* The term "maternal floor infarction" is a misnomer.[31] The lesion does not represent infarction. It is characterized by excessive fibrin deposition in the decidua basalis and in the adjacent intervillous space.

2. *Gross features.* The maternal surface of the placenta has a thickened, yellowish-white appearance.
3. *Histologic features.* The villi near the maternal surface are enmeshed in a large amount of fibrin (Figure 45). Severe fibrin deposition may involve all or a large part of the placenta in some cases. This results in reduction of blood flow through these intervillous spaces and eventually in sclerotic, avascular villi.
4. *Significance.* Abortion or stillbirths are the fetal complications.
5. *Pathogenesis.* It is not known. Fox[4] considers this lesion as a sequela and not as a cause of intrauterine fetal death.

Robb et al.[32] demonstrated herpes simplex virus (HSV) antigen in the cytoplasm of choriodecidual cells and Hofbauer cells of villi at the maternal surface by immunoperoxidase stain in five of eight cases of maternal floor infarction. No overt HSV infection was demonstrated in the fetus, and a maternal history of HSV infection was lacking. They suggested that maternal floor infarctions may be related to latent HSV infection. Maternal floor infarction may recur in subsequent pregnancies.[31]

Villitis

Villitis can be acute or chronic. It may have a focal or diffuse distribution and may vary in severity from mild to moderate to severe. Acute villitis is seen primarily when organisms reach the placenta via the maternal blood. Spread of organisms from adjacent basal endometrium may also occur. The infection may eventually spread from the villi to the membranes. In rare instances the organisms may reach the villi via the fetal circulation, which is invaded by organisms reaching the fetal tissues through aspiration or ingestion of infected amniotic fluid. The barrier to infection is provided by the placental cells and

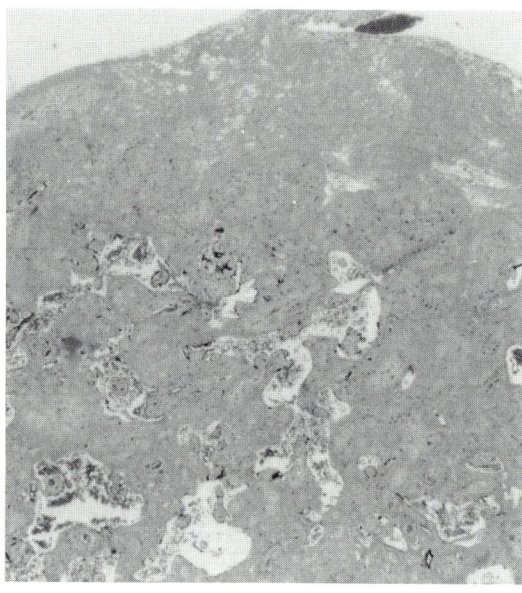

FIGURE 45. Maternal floor infarction characterized by severe fibrin deposition between the villi near the maternal surface (H&E, ×40).

tissues (the trophoblast, its basement membrane, stroma and Hofbauer cells of the villi, and endothelium and basement membrane of the villous capillaries) through which the organisms must pass to produce placental and subsequently fetal infection. In humans, the placental barrier does not appear to be very efficient since a large number of organisms can cross it. The organisms may break the barrier by causing injury to and death of the placental cells, either directly or by producing a toxin or inciting an inflammatory response which produces cellular damage. Receptors for viruses (e.g., CD4 receptors for HIV) may be present on the cells of the placenta, enabling attachment and entry of the virus into the placental cells and subsequently into the fetus.

The following types of villitis have been described by Altshuler and Russell:[33]

1. *Proliferative villitis characterized by chronic inflammatory infiltration of the villi (lymphocytes, plasma cells, histiocytes)* (Figure 46). This type of villitis is seen in rubella, CMV infection, and syphilis. The placenta in these infections is bulky and pale on gross examination (Figure 47). Organisms (e.g., CMV, *Treponema pallidum*) can be demonstrated by routine and special stains (Figure 48).
2. *Necrotizing villitis with necrosis of villi and an acute inflammatory infiltrate.* This type of villitis is seen as a result of hematogenous spread of bacteria. *Listeria monocytogenes* is the most common cause of necrotizing villitis (Figure 49), but it may also be seen in acute viral infections.
3. *Granulomatous villitis with formation of granulomas (central necrosis, lymphohistiocytic infiltrate, and multinucleated giant cells).* This type of villitis is seen in toxoplasmosis (Figures 50, 51), syphilis, and tuberculosis.
4. *Reparative villitis with formation of granulation tissue, fibroblastic proliferation, and fibrosis.* This type of villitis represents a later stage of active villitis.
5. *Stromal fibrosis.* This represents the end stage of various forms of villitis

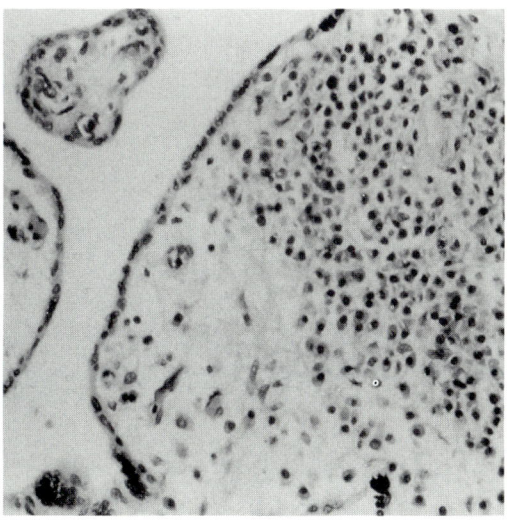

FIGURE 46. Proliferative villitis, characterized by lymphoplasmacytic and histiocytic infiltration of the villi (H&E, ×250).

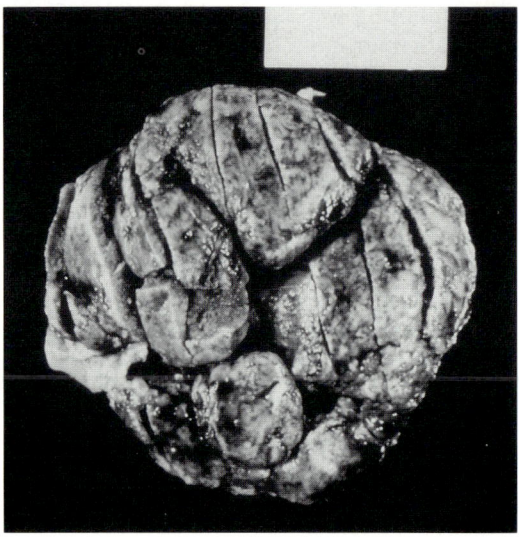

FIGURE 47. Large, pale, bulky placenta in toxoplasmosis.

outlined above. The villi show fibrosis and marked hypovascularity or avascularity. Occasional chronic inflammatory cells may be present.

Chronic Intervillositis

When villitis is present, the inflammatory infiltrate may extend to the intervillous space as a result of ulceration of the trophoblastic lining. However, an inflammatory infiltrate in the intervillous space may also occur in the absence of villitis. This lesion is labeled "chronic intervillositis (CIV)." CIV characterized by the presence of mononuclear cell infiltration (histiocytes and lymphocytes) admixed with rare neutrophils in the intervillous space has been described by

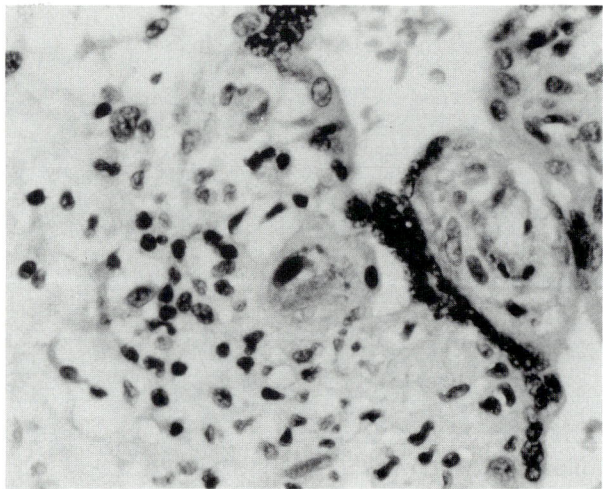

FIGURE 48. CMV inclusions in a stromal cell of the villus in CMV villitis. Note the mildly lymphomononuclear infiltrate (H&E, ×400).

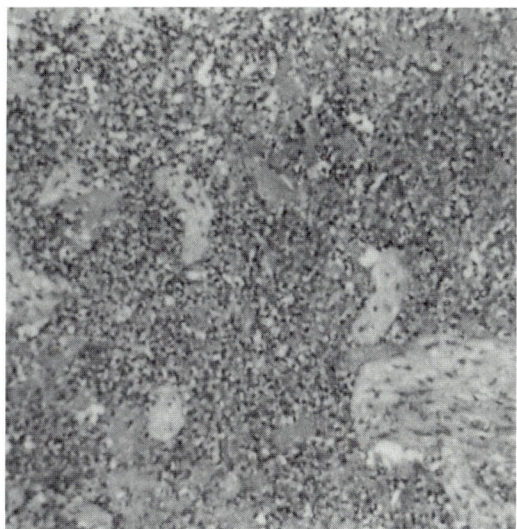

FIGURE 49. Acute necrotizing villitis with microabscess formation in listeriosis. *L. monocytogenes* was cultured from and demonstrated by Gram stain of the placenta. (H&E, ×250.)

Jacques and Qureshi.[34] Intervillous inflammatory cells of maternal origin, as well as prominent intravillous and perivillous fibrinoid depositions, are also present. Vasculitis may be present in both villitis and CIV (Figure 52). There was death of the fetus or of the neonate in five of the six cases of CIV reported by Jacques and Qureshi. Maternal conditions seen in five of these six cases included preeclampsia, hypertension, substance abuse, systemic lupus erythematosus and diabetes. The etiology of CIV is not known. Immunologic factors or infection have been suggested as possible etiologic factors.

Bacterial Villitis

As indicated above, enteric and other Gram-negative organisms and group B streptococci can conceivably produce necrotizing villitis as a consequence of

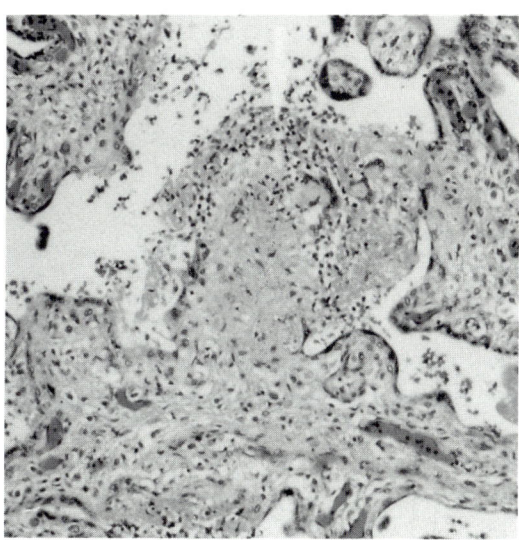

FIGURE 50. Granulomatous villitis with necrosis, a lymphomononuclear infiltrate, and giant cells in toxoplasmosis (H&E, ×100).

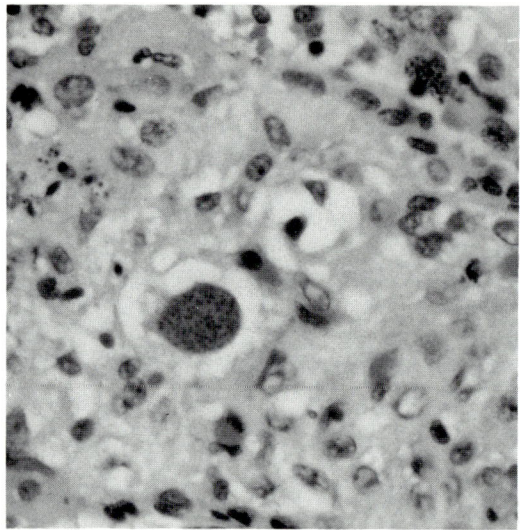

FIGURE 51. Toxoplasma cyst in granulomatous villitis (H&E, ×400).

maternal septicemia. However, septicemia due to bacteria such as staphylococci, group B streptococci, and enteric and other Gram-negative organisms is unusual during pregnancy, the more common route of transmission of these organisms being the ascending route from the maternal genital tract. Therefore, chorioamnionitis is the more common type of placental lesion related to these organisms (see the section on acute chorioamnionitis below). Bacterial villitis when present can usually be recognized histologically since abundant organisms are present in the foci of necrosis and inflammation.[33]

Listeria monocytogenes. These small, Gram-positive bacilli are ubiquitous and contaminate milk, cheese, vegetables, and meat. The organisms spread to the

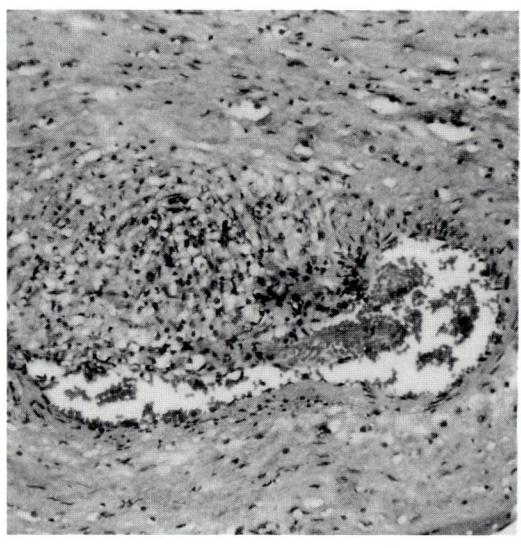

FIGURE 52. Vasculitis of a villous blood vessel in villitis (H&E, ×250).

placenta by the hematogenous route or by the ascending route from the maternal genital tract. Whether one or the other route is more common is not known. However, some investigators have suggested that the ascending route is the primary route of transmission to the placenta and that necrotizing villitis may be secondary to fetal septicemia.[35] The pharynx and gastrointestinal tract are the main portals of entry of the organisms in the mother. Maternal genital tract colonization probably occurs via fecal contamination. Gastroenteritis, a flu-like syndrome and septicemia due to *L. monocytogenes* occurring in the mother predispose to the spread of the organisms to the placenta (and to the fetus). The placenta shows small, yellowish, necrotic foci on gross examination. Histologically, microabscesses are noted in these foci (Figure 49). Chorioamnionitis is also present in *L. monocytogenes* infection. The fetus may show widespread necrotic lesions with or without an inflammatory reaction in the lungs, liver, adrenals, spleen, bone marrow, and meninges. Arteritis is also present in the various organs. Gram stain readily reveals the Gram-positive bacilli in the foci of villitis and in the fetal tissues.

Treponema pallidum. The placenta in congenital syphilis (CS) tends to be large and pale. Focal villitis characterized by a predominantly plasmacytic infiltrate is present. In some cases, chronic lymphohistiocytic infiltration is present in the villi. Granulomatous inflammation may also occur. Endarteritis, intimal and perivascular fibrous proliferation and perivascular inflammation are characteristically seen in the arteries of the stem villi. Organisms can be demonstrated in the foci of villitis by silver stain. Villous immaturity may be present. Necrotizing funisitis has been described in CS.[36] (see the section on lesions of the umbilical cord below). Plasmacytic deciduitis is frequently present. In some cases of documented maternal syphilis, the placenta may appear normal.

In recent years there has been a resurgence of maternal syphilis and CS, particularly in the inner cities. In New York City alone, there was a fivefold increase in the number of cases of CS between 1986 and 1988. The lack of prenatal care in many of the mothers suffering from syphilis may result in delay in the diagnosis of CS. In such cases, the histologic findings in the placenta are helpful in suggesting the possibility of CS, with confirmation obtained by the demonstration of organisms by silver stain and/or serology.

Mycobacterium tuberculosis. Placental tuberculosis is rare in Western countries. Hematogenous spread of the organisms results in miliary tubercles in the placenta. Caseating granulomas may also be seen in the decidua.[37,38]

Mycoplasma and chlamydia infections. There is usually chorioamnionitis in mycoplasma infection. Dische et al.[39] have also described acute villitis with neutrophilic infiltration and focal loss of trophoblast in two cases. No placental lesion has been attributed to chlamydia.

Viral Villitis
1. *Rubella and CMV.* These are the most important viral causes of villitis. In rubella, the following types of lesions are seen in the acute stage: (a) focal necrotizing villitis with endarteritis of the villous blood vessels or (b) focal trophoblastic necrosis with or without neutrophilic infiltration and perivil-

lous fibrin deposition. Eosinophilic inclusions may be present in the endothelial cells or trophoblast.[40,41] There are increased numbers of Hofbauer cells. Perivasculitis is seen commonly. In the chronic stage of rubella, the villi are avascular and fibrotic. Active lesions may be present concurrently. In symptomatic CMV infection of the infant, placental lesions are present in the majority of cases. The diagnostic feature of the lesion is the presence of characteristic intranuclear viral inclusions in enlarged endothelial and stromal cells (Figure 48). Cytoplasmic inclusions may also be present. The CMV inclusion can be identified specifically by immunoperoxidase stain. Necrotizing, proliferative and reparative types of villitis can also occur.[42] Inflammatory cells include lymphocytes, plasma cells and histiocytes (Figure 46). The inflammatory infiltrate may extend into the intervillous space. Multinucleated giant cells may be present occasionally. Villous edema and calcification of the stroma and basement membrane have been described.

2. *Vaccinia.* Focal necrotizing villitis has been described in vaccinia infection of the placenta, which is a complication of vaccination during pregnancy.[40]

3. *Variola minor.* Rare cases of necrotizing granulomatous villitis have been reported in variola minor (a mild form of smallpox occurring previously in South America and western Africa).

4. *Varicella.* In varicella, villitis is characterized by necrosis, neutrophilic infiltration and granuloma formation.[43] There are no viral inclusions in the placental tissue, although inclusions were present in the decidual cells in the cases described by Garcia.[43]

5. *Herpes simplex virus (HSV).* HSV usually spreads via the maternal genital tract. Therefore, chorioamnionitis, which may be related to concomitant bacterial infection, is the more common lesion. Intranuclear HSV inclusions may be present in the amniotic epithelium. HSV inclusions can be identified specifically by immunoperoxidase stain.[44] In rare cases of hematogenous spread of HSV, there is focal necrosis of villi with a paucity or absence of an inflammatory reaction and the presence of inclusion-like bodies in the syncytiotrophoblast.

    Lymphoplasmacytic infiltrates in the umbilical cord, decidua, and chorionic plate have been described in some cases.[45,46] Schwartz and Caldwell demonstrated a positive reaction for HSV in the decidual cells by using the DNA in situ hybridization technique.[47] Typical inclusions of HSV or an inflammatory reaction were not seen in the decidua. Hyde and Giacoia have reported the occurrence of HSV inclusions and/or positive staining on immunoperoxidase stain in the subamniotic mesenchymal cells of the umbilical cord.[46]

6. *Infectious mononucleosis.* In abortions occurring in maternal infectious mononucleosis, villitis with lymphoplasmacytic infiltration and necrosis of trophoblastic cells has been described.[48] It is not certain whether these lesions were related to Epstein–Barr virus.[48]

7. *Coxsackie and ECHO viruses.* These can infect the fetus. Villitis with or without necrosis, intervillositis and massive intervillous fibrin deposits have been described in rare instances.

8. *Poliomyelitis, mumps, influenza, and parainfluenza viruses.* Placental lesions have not been described in these infections.
9. *Hepatitis viruses.* Fetal infection occurs rarely in maternal hepatitis. A. Placental pathology has not been described. In hepatitis B, the surface antigen (HBsAg) has been demonstrated in the Hofbauer cells and endothelial cells of the villi in placentas of asymptomatic carriers by immunohistologic methods.[49] No pathologic changes except for the presence of bilirubin in the Hofbauer cells and focal syncytiotrophoblast necrosis are present when the mother suffers from hepatitis.
10. *Human parvovirus infection (HPV).* The characteristic feature is the presence of eosinophilic intranuclear inclusions in the normoblasts in the villous capillaries, which are detected by histology and electron microscopy (Figures 53 and 54).[50,51] The placenta is frequently hydropic. Necrosis and calcification of villi may occur.[5] Prominent erythroblasts may be present in the villous capillaries.

In a series of five cases of proven HPV infection of the fetus, diagnostic inclusions were found in the placenta in only two.[52] Thus negative placental findings do not necessarily rule out fetal infection. Mark et al.[53] used polymerase chain reaction (PCR) to demonstrate HPV infection of fetal tissues. These

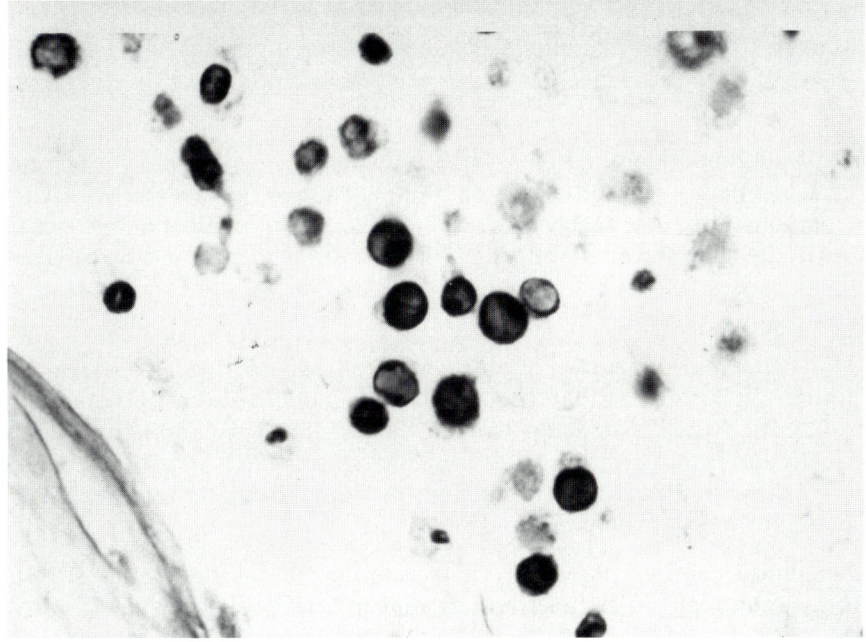

FIGURE 53. Intranuclear eosinophilic inclusions in the normoblasts of bone marrow in a fetus infected by human parvovirus. Similar inclusions were seen in the fetal normoblasts in placental capillaries (H&E, ×400).

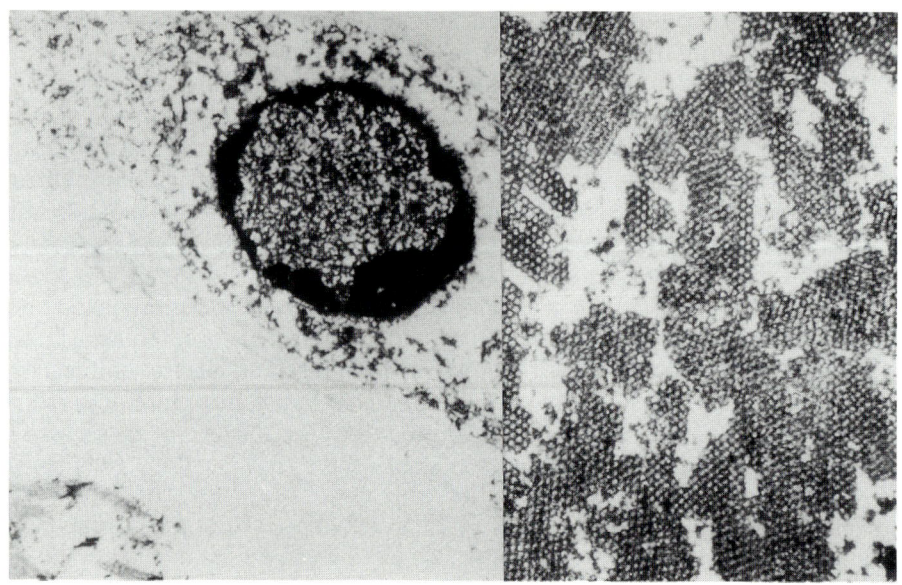

FIGURE 54. Left panel: Electron micrograph of a normoblast showing an intranuclear viral inclusion (uranyl acetate and lead citrate, ×10,000). Right panel: Parvovirus, showing its crystalline structure (×58,000). (Courtesy of Dr. Alexander S. Knisely)

investigators found that histologic examination of fetal tissues was as sensitive as the PCR technique. Placental tissue was not included in this comparative study.

Human Immunodeficiency Virus (HIV) Infection

Perinatal pathology of HIV infection has been reviewed recently.[54] HIV has been demonstrated by morphologic or molecular biologic methods and/or culture in the maternal genital tract and its secretions, placenta, amniotic fluid, and fetal tissues (thymus, lung, brain, spleen). The reader is referred to the review article[54] for details of references.

Maternal Genital Tract. Chronic cervicitis characterized by mononuclear cell infiltration and lymphoid aggregates in the mucosa and/or submucosa has been described in HIV-infected women. Isolation of HIV from these biopsy specimens and from vaginal and cervical secretions of HIV-infected women, as well as the presence of HIV antigens in the mononuclear cells, endothelial cells and lymphocytes, has been reported.

Placenta. Jauniaux and co-workers[55] studied 49 placentas, 7 fetuses and 2 stillbirths from central African and European HIV-positive women with or without fully developed AIDS. No villitis was noted in the placenta, but irrespective of gestational age, the villi were coarse, cellular and hypovascularized. There was a high incidence of chorioamnionitis (42%). Ultrastructural studies revealed isolated retrovirus-like particles with some morphologic similarities to HIV (100 nM in size, with a dense central or eccentric core) in the syncytiotrophoblast, fibroblasts, and endothelial cells of villous capillaries and free membranes in 5 of the 13 placentas. The authors pointed out that the viral particles seen in their cases also resembled the type c viral particles described in the syncytiotrophoblast of normal human term placenta. More recently, Chandwani et al.[56] have demonstrated HIV p24 antigen and nucleic acids in the trophoblast by the immunoperoxidase method and in situ hybridization in 2 of 20 (10%) term placentas from HIV-infected mothers. Chorioamnionitis was seen in 60% of the 43 placentas examined histologically. Martin et al.[57] found positive staining for p24 by the immunoperoxidase method in the Hofbauer cells, vascular endothelium and intermediate trophoblasts in four of nine (44%) placentas from HIV-positive women.

Receptors for HIV (i.e., CD4) are present on the trophoblastic and stromal cells of the chorionic villi and endothelial cells of the placental blood vessels.[58] HIV infection of first-trimester placental tissue has been shown in the organ culture.[58] In contrast to these positive findings, absence of HIV proteins by the immunohistochemical method and of nucleic acids by in situ hybridization in placentas from HIV-infected women has also been reported. There is one report in which HIV was cultured from the placenta of an asymptomatic, HIV-positive mother. The details of how contamination with maternal blood was avoided at the time of obtaining placental material were not given. The authors commented that the positive culture was probably the result of positive maternal blood culture.

Amniotic Fluid. There is one case report in which HIV was cultured from and HIV antigens were demonstrated in amniotic fluid and cells.

Fetal Tissues. The presence of HIV reverse transcriptase activity and antigens in various organs (thymus, brain, lung and spleen) from a 15- and a 20-week fetus has been demonstrated by in situ hybridization, immunofluorescence, and the polymerase chain reaction (PCR) technique. Viral DNA was demonstrated in fetal tissues (thymus and spleen) in about 75% of the cases even when attempts at viral cultures from these tissues were unsuccessful. Attempts to culture HIV from cord blood from fetuses of HIV-positive mothers have been unsuccessful.

Pathologic Features of HIV-Positive Fetal Tissues. There is no mention of any pathologic findings or of any pathologic study of the fetal tissues in most of the reports discussed. Focal lymphocytic depletion, infiltration by CD4-positive macrophages, increased density of epithelial cells and thickening of the lobular septa have been reported in HIV-positive fetal thymuses.

Mechanism and Timing of Fetal Infection. The results described above indicate that there are HIV receptors on the cells in normal placentas (trophoblast, endothelium, stromal cells) and that these cells are infectable by HIV. The frequency of HIV infection of the placenta varies from 0 to 44% in different series. The presence of HIV in the fetal tissues has been shown after 15 weeks' gestation. Fetal specimens from earlier gestations have not been tested. The brain and CD4 lymphocytes in the thymus and spleen have been the primary sites of localization of HIV in the fetus. Cells expressing the CD4 marker are detected in the thymus by 11 weeks' gestation. Therefore infection of fetal tissues is unlikely before 11 weeks' gestation.

Besides the infection of the placenta, followed by that of the fetal tissues, other mechanisms of HIV transmission to the fetus include passive transfer during the maternal viremic phase, passage of infected CD4 lymphocytes from the mother, and active transport of HIV-immunoglobulin G complex. It should be noted that in none of the known fetal infections (CMV, toxoplasmosis, syphilis, rubella, etc.) does passive transfer without infection of the placenta occur. The only possible exception is HPV infection.

The low frequency of viral localization in the placenta and fetal tissues in some of reported series may be due to the low frequency of intrauterine transplacental maternofetal transmission of HIV in early pregnancy or to the low sensitivity of the techniques other than PCR. The presence of HIV in the secretions and tissues of the maternal genital tract and the exposure of fetus to maternal blood during delivery support the intrapartum transmission of HIV. The failure of HIV localization by in situ hybridization and PCR in 10 of 12 fetuses of HIV-positive mothers reported recently by Ehrnst et al.[59] supports perinatal (i.e., at the time of delivery) HIV transmission as the more frequent mode. It is of interest to note that maternofetal transmission of HIV has been observed in a chimpanzee.

Placental Barrier. Morphologically, the placental barrier consists of trophoblast and its basement membrane, mesenchymal tissue including macrophages (Hofbauer cells) of the villus, endothelium, capillary basement membrane and vasculosyncytial membrane. The placental barrier may normally be effective in preventing viral transmission. But concurrent placental inflammation may compromise the integrity of the placental barrier. Thus, the presence of other placental infections such as chorioamnionitis or syphilis may enhance the perinatal transmission of HIV. Ischemia and vascular insufficiency may also result in breaks in the placental barrier. It has also been suggested that interaction between HIV-infected maternal lymphocytes and the syncytiotrophoblast may lead to internalization of HIV by the syncytiotrophoblast via an endocytic process.

Fungal Infection

Chorioamnionitis and funisitis are the characteristic lesions seen in Candida infection.[5] In a case of abortion due to candidiasis focal necrosis of villi with intervillous abscesses and chronic villitis have been described.[60] Placental infarcts and necrotizing villitis with perivillous fibrin deposition occur in maternal coccidioidomycosis.[61] The spherules of *Coccidioides immitis* can be demonstrated in the lesions. Kida et al[62] have described presence of colonies of cryptococcus species in the intervillous spaces in the placenta from a woman with AIDS who died of disseminated cryptococcosis. There were no organisms in the villi nor was there evidence of villitis.

Parasitic Infection

Transplacental transmission of *Trypanosoma cruzi* infection (Chagas' disease occurring in South America) has been described.[63] Large numbers of organisms are seen in the Hofbauer cells. Chronic villitis with granulomatous reaction and fibrosis is present. Intervillous spaces show fibrin deposition and accumulation of mononuclear cells. Schistosomiasis occurring in Far East and Africa can involve the placenta. Ova may be present in the villi and/or the intervillous spaces. Inflammatory reaction is usually absent. Congenital malaria has been described in tropical countries with endemic incidence of the infection. The organisms can be demonstrated in the smears made from the placenta and in the maternal RBCs in the intervillous spaces (Figure 55). Collections of macrophages and fibrin deposition are also seen in these spaces. Abundant malarial pigment (derived from breakdown of hemoglobin) deposited in these macrophages, fibrin, and the villi imparts a dark brown to black color to the placenta. Lymphomononuclear infiltration of the villi may be present. Plasmodia have not been demonstrated in the villi, and it is not clear how the organisms spread across the placenta. It appears that it occurs via the transfer of maternal blood to the fetus—a phenomenon that is rare.[5]

Toxoplasma gondii is the most important parasitic placental infection in Western countries. The placenta shows involvement of varying severity.[64] There may be (1) mild lymphoplasmacytic infiltration of villi, (2) granulomatous lesions characterized by foci of villous necrosis with mononuclear and giant cells (Figure 50), or (3) necrotizing villitis with acute inflammatory reaction. Although both free and encysted forms of the organisms can be present, the latter are more common (Figure 51).

Villitis of Unknown Etiology

The presence of inflammatory infiltration of villi can occur without any demonstrable infectious etiology. Altshuler[65] labeled this entity "villitis of unknown etiology (VUE)." VUE has an incidence of 5–8% in consecutively examined placentas. VUE may be focal or diffuse. Focal VUE can be easily overlooked if all the slides of the placenta are not scanned carefully. Foci of "hypercellular" villi should raise the suspicion of VUE. Lack of interobserver concordance among experienced pathologists has been reported recently by

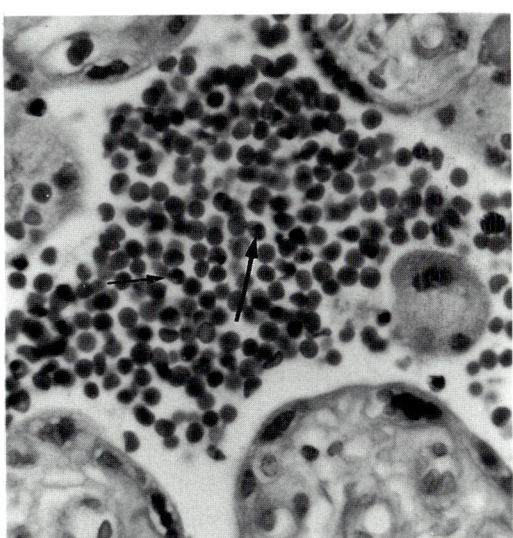

FIGURE 55. Malarial parasites in the RBCs in the intervillous space in maternal malaria (H&E, ×400).

Khong et al.[66] The extent of histologic sampling of the placenta will also affect the frequency of diagnosis of VUE. The whole range of inflammatory reactions described above in relation to the types of villitis can be exhibited by VUE, but most commonly there is a lymphohistiocytic infiltration of the villi (Figure 56). Plasma cells are not seen in VUE. Degenerative changes in the villi in the vicinity of an infarct may resemble VUE. Such changes should not be confused with VUE. Lymphocytic infiltration of decidua is present frequently.[67] VUE can be recurrent.[68]

The most significant clinical correlate of VUE is intrauterine growth retardation (IUGR). The incidence of ischemia in the placenta which shows VUE is also high.[69] The severity of placental ischemia, not of VUE, correlates with the severity of IUGR. Infants with IUGR apparently do not show subsequent impairment. However, long-term follow-up studies are lacking. Other clinical correlates include a high incidence of congenital anomalies and perinatal morbidity and mortality. These clinical abnormalities have a higher incidence in recurrent VUE.[68] The following three possible etiologies of VUE have been suggested:[5] (1) it is a viral infection, (2) it represents an attempt at rejection of the placental graft, or (3) it is related to preeclampsia and infarcts. However, it should be noted that the villous changes in preeclampsia and around an infarct are primarily of the degenerative type. Therefore, the last theory may not be valid. The inflammatory cells in VUE consist of activated macrophages and T-helper lymphocytes, suggesting that it is an immunologic lesion.[70] In a recent study in which in-situ hybridization using X and Y chromosome specific probes was performed on four placentas from male infants showing VUE, Redline and Patterson[70a] have shown that majority of the T cells in the villous inflammatory infiltrate were of maternal origin (xx cells). These results are suggestive of maternal immunologic reaction playing a role in the pathogenesis of VUE.[70a,70b]

Tumors of the Placenta

Gestational trophoblastic diseases (partial and complete hydatiform moles, invasive hydatidiform mole, choriocarcinoma, placental site trophoblastic tu-

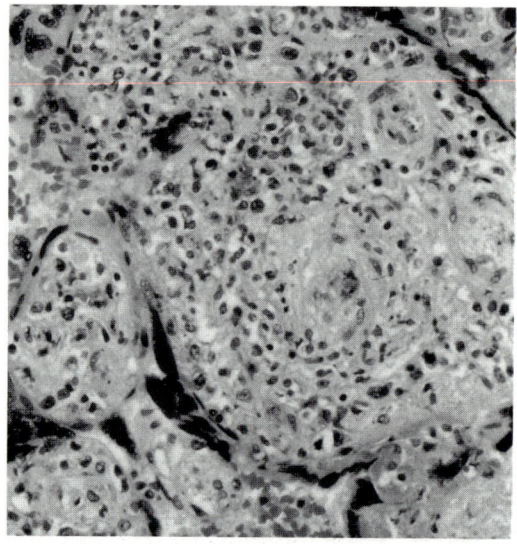

FIGURE 56. Villitis of unknown etiology characterized by lymphohistiocytic infiltration of the villi (H&E, ×250).

mor, miscellaneous lesions such as exaggerated placental site, placental site nodule and unclassified trophoblastic lesion), which generally fall into the realm of gynecologic pathology,[71,72] are not discussed in this book. Only the nontrophoblastic tumors are described. There are two types of primary nontrophoblastic tumors of the placental parenchyma: hemangioma (chorangioma or chorioangioma) and teratoma. Metastasis of maternal and fetal tumors to the placenta can also occur.[73]

Hemangioma

Hemangiomas that are considered malformative rather than neoplastic lesions usually are single small lesions. Careful examination of thin slices of the placenta is necessary to detect these lesions. A large, nodular, red-tan mass protruding on the fetal surface or replacing a portion of the cotyledon on the maternal surface or with a pedicle may be seen occasionally (Figure 57). Diffuse hemangiomatous involvement of the placenta (hemangiomatosis) is extremely rare. Histologically, the tumor shows capillary-like or cavernous vascular channels embedded in stroma of variable quantity (Figure 58). Necrosis, hyalinization, calcification and myxoid change can occur. Small hemangiomas are of no clinical significance. However, the larger tumors are associated with increased weight of the placenta (possibly due to stasis secondary to compression), polyhydramnios, antepartum hemorrhage (due to abruptio placentae or directly from the tumor), IUGR, fetal cardiomegaly and neonatal anemia, edema, and thrombocytopenia.

Teratoma

Teratomas of the placenta are extremely rare. The well-circumscribed, solid tumor is located on the fetal surface between the amnion and chorion or in the membranes at the placental margin. These tumors are composed of various mature epithelial, neural, and mesenchymal elements. A placental tumor composed of glycogen-containing polygonal cells resembling hepatocytes, with focal

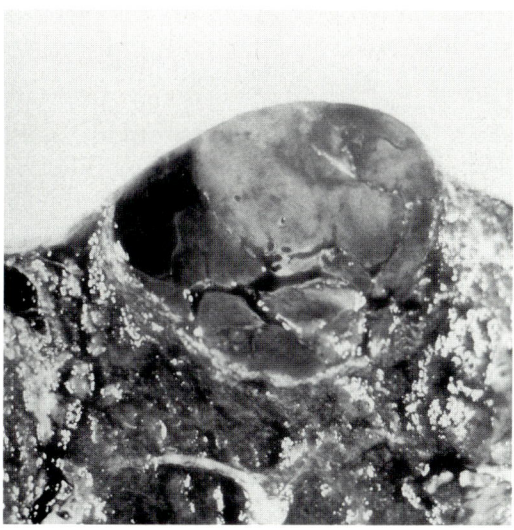

FIGURE 57. Hemangioma of the placenta characterized by a fleshy tan, brown, firm, solid-appearing nodule.

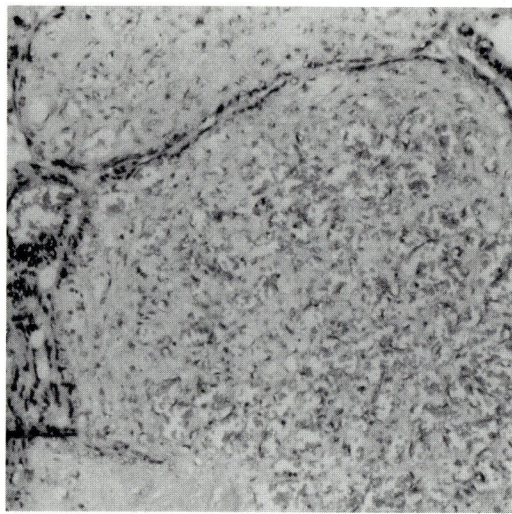

FIGURE 58. Hemangioma of the placenta showing proliferation of capillary-type vessels in expanded villous-like structures (H&E, ×100).

reactivity to alpha fetoprotein and α-antitrypsin and presence of bile canaliculi on electron microscopy, has been described by Chen et al.[74] They suggested that this hepatocellular adenoma represented a monodermal teratoma. Germ cells may show aberrant migration into the umbilical cord through the gut, which normally evaginates into the base of the cord during early fetal development. These germ cells may continue to migrate farther to the fetal surface of the placenta, giving rise to teratomas. Teratomas can arise from these misplaced germ cells.

Metastatic Tumors

Placental metastases have been described in maternal neoplastic disorders such as leukemia, malignant lymphoma, melanoma, carcinomas of the breast, rectum, and lung, and Ewing's sarcoma. A brown or black nodule of metastatic melanoma may be seen grossly. Metastasis of other neoplastic disorders may not be demonstrable on gross examination. Histologic examination reveals that in most instances the metastatic tumor is confined to the intervillous space. However, in occasional cases, invasion of the villous stroma and capillaries can occur. Metastasis to fetal organs has been described in malignant melanoma. Placental involvement in fetal tumors has been described in cases of neuroblastoma, melanoma, hepatoblastoma, and leukemia. The placenta is large, heavy and pale in neuroblastoma. The malignant cells are confined to the capillaries of the villi. In leukemia, infiltration of villous stroma can occur.

LESIONS OF THE UMBILICAL CORD

The umbilical cord has two arteries and a vein, which are embedded in Wharton's jelly, composed of mucoid ground substance and a network of fibroblasts. Wharton's jelly protects the blood vessels from mechanical trauma. The umbilical cord is covered by amniotic epithelium. The umbilical artery has two layers of muscle coat that are contracted by giving an undulating outline to its luminal surface in histologic sections. The umbilical vein shows a well-defined internal elastic lamina. (Umbilical arteries do not show such a lamina). The umbilical vessels are arranged in a spiral fashion within the umbilical cord. Absence of umbilical cord (achordia) is extremely rare and is seen in severely malformed abortuses.

Short and Long Umbilical Cords

The length of the umbilical cord often cannot be assessed accurately by the pathologist because a segment of the cord may be retained in the delivery room. It is therefore imperative that the length be recorded on the surgical requisition form by the delivery room personnel. Cord length may vary from ~32 cm at 20–21 weeks' gestation to ~59 cm at term.[75] It has been estimated that a length of 32 cm would prevent cord traction at normal vertex delivery. Therefore a cord <32 cm in length at any gestational age is considered a short umbilical cord. Short cord length may be a consequence of decreased fetal movement. It may not produce any fetal morbidity. However, excessive traction on the cord during delivery may lead to interference with the umbilical vascular circulation or to rupture, with consequent fetal distress.[76] Naeye[75] reported a correlation of short umbilical cord with subsequent low IQ values and neurologic abnormalities. An umbilical cord measuring >70 cm is considered long.[77] An abnormally long cord is prone to formation of knots, prolapse, or compression leading to fetal distress or death. Large infants tend to have long cords. The precise pathogenesis of abnormal cord length is not known.

Single Umbilical Artery (SUA)

The incidence of SUA varies from 0.2 to 1.1%. SUA may be missed unless careful gross examination and histologic examination of well-oriented cross sections from the relatively nonspiral segments of the cord are done. One of the two umbilical arteries may be totally absent (primary aplasia), or its atrophic remnants may be found on histologic examination. There is a high incidence (25–50%) of congenital anomalies such as renal dysplasia or agenesis, tracheo-esophageal fistula and CNS malformations in the fetus with SUA.

Supernumerary Umbilical Vessels

This abnormality has not been fully investigated. A tortuous portion of an umbilical blood vessel may be cut in more than one plane in a cross section, giving a spurious impression of supernumerary blood vessels. However, occurrence of true supernumerary arteries and veins has been reported. It has been suggested that the supernumerary blood vessels may be vitelline in origin. Alternatively, there may be persistence of the right umbilical vein that normally disappears during development. There is no high incidence of congenital anomalies in fetuses with supernumerary umbilical vessels.

Varices and Aneurysms

Varices of the vein and aneurysms of the arteries are rare. These lesions can be seen in the blood vessels of the umbilical cord and/or of the fetal surface of the placenta. Bleeding from or thrombosis in these lesions may occur. Aneurysms may be associated with SUA. Thrombi in the aneurysms may be associated with

IUGR and maternal diabetes. Aneurysms are considered congenital anomalies (Figure 59). The occurrence of the aneurysms may be suspected during pregnancy by abnormalities of blood flow detected on Doppler ultrasound studies. The varices should be distinguished from chorionic cysts with hemorrhage within them. Angiomatous malformation of the blood vessels of the chorionic plate consisting of multiple tangled blood vessels has been described recently by Sander.[77a]

Thrombosis of Umbilical Blood Vessels

Thrombosis is usually a secondary phenomenon associated with umbilical cord abnormalities such as cord compression (e.g., in velamentous insertion), knot formation, entanglement in amniotic bands, stricture, torsion, long cord, short cord, trauma due to intrauterine transfusion, varices, and aneurysms. Obstetrical complications such as malpresentation, multiple gestation, precipitate delivery, and abdominal trauma and maternal disease (e.g., diabetes) and fetal conditions (hydrops fetalis, fetomaternal hemorrhage, etc.) may also be associated with thrombosis. In rare cases, no predisposing cause can be found. Venous thrombi are more common than arterial thrombi. The incidence of thrombosis is higher in high-risk gestations. Old thrombi may become calcified. Severe fetal sequelae, including fetal death related to occlusion of the lumen of the thrombosed vessel, may ensue.

Hematoma and Rupture of Umbilical Blood Vessels

Blood is drawn from the umbilical cord vessels by the delivery personnel or neonatologist, which might lead to formation of small hemorrhages or hematomas of the cord due to leakage. The amount of blood lost in such instances is inconsequential. Pathologic hematomas due to rupture, with varying amounts of hemorrhage, are seen in association with velamentous insertion of the cord,

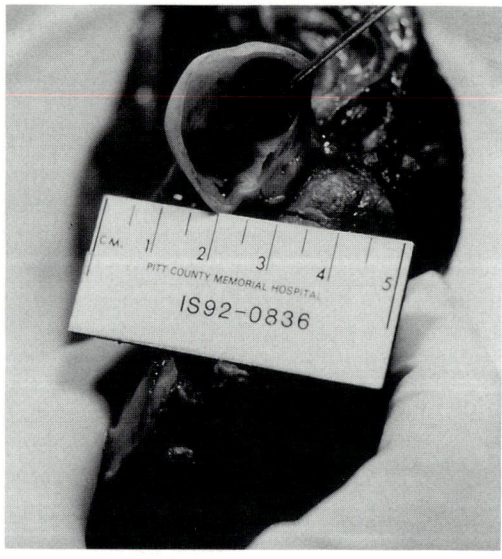

FIGURE 59. Aneurysm of a branch of the umbilical artery of the fetal surface of the placenta.

short umbilical cord, aneurysms, and varices, and as a complication of amniocentesis and intrauterine intravascular transfusion. The amount of blood lost from rupture of the cord cannot be estimated by the pathologist. The hematoma occurring in association with the aforementioned lesions should be measured and the amount of blood carefully estimated. Severe blood loss from such lesions leads to fetal morbidity and even mortality.

Calcification of Umbilical Blood Vessels

This lesion is rare. Calcification can involve the vessel wall or the lumen. In the former, there is also sclerosis of the vessel wall, and calcification may extend to the Wharton jelly area. The etiology is not known, but intrauterine infection has been implicated because of the concomitant presence of inflammation in the cord, membranes and decidua in some cases.[78] Luminal calcification represents calcification of an old thrombus.

Abnormal Insertion of the Umbilical Cord

The umbilical cord is normally inserted on the fetal surface of the placenta, at or close to its center. Marginal insertion (Battledore placenta) also occurs. In velamentous insertion, the cord inserts on the membranes. The umbilical blood vessels unprotected by the Wharton jelly course over the membranes. These vessels are therefore prone to rupture and compression during delivery, resulting in significant fetal distress. Thrombosis may also occur. Such complications are more likely when the blood vessels lie across the internal os of the cervix (vasa previa). Velamentous insertion is more frequent in placentas with SUA and twin placentas. IUGR may occur in fetuses with velamentous insertion of their umbilical cords. A section for histologic examination should be taken from the velamentous insertion site for permanent documentation of the lesion. The incidence of marginal and velamentous insertions is higher in stillbirths than in normal infants.[79] Marginal insertion is also reported to be more common in abortions, malformed fetuses, and neonatal asphyxia. In furcate insertion, the vessels lose their protective covering of Wharton's jelly proximal to their insertion on the fetal surface of the placenta. Thrombosis, compression, and rupture can occur in furcate insertion. The pathogenesis of abnormal insertion is not known.

Knots in the Umbilical Cord

There are two types of knots: (1) *false knots*—nodular swellings of the umbilical cord produced by segmental redundancy, ectasia, or branching of the blood vessels or focal excessive accumulation of Wharton's jelly (false knots have no clinical significance) and (2) *true knots*—knots prone to occur in excessively long cords. The tightness of the cord determines the presence of vascular complications such as edema, congestion, and thrombosis. The normal blood pressure in the umbilical vein is 10 mmHg. In in vitro experiments, a pressure of 100–110 mmHg is required to overcome the resistance in a tight knot caused by a 100-g weight.[80] Thus the fetus is deprived of umbilical venous blood when the knots are sufficiently tight. True knots are associated with a perinatal mortality rate of 8–11%.[4]

The umbilical cord showing a true knot should be carefuly assessed grossly and histologically for changes in the umbilical vein, which may be markedly dilated and congested on the placental side. There may be thrombotic occlusion of the umbilical vein, and the cord may be edematous. Sections of the cord through the knot and either side should be taken for histologic examination. In the absence of evidence of obstruction to umbilical venous flow, the knot is considered to be clinically insignificant.

Torsion of the Umbilical Cord

The normal cord is spiraled, usually in the counterclockwise direction. It has been suggested that the spiraling is caused by fetal movements. Excessive spiraling has been considered to be a cause of intrauterine fetal death by some investigators. In torsion there is excessive rigid, localized spiraling of the cord, usually at the fetal end.[76] Some investigators consider localized narrowing (stricture, coarctation) of excessively spiraled umbilical cord to be synonymous with torsion.[5] The pathogenesis of torsion is not known. A cord stricture (see below) and long cord predispose to torsion. There is obstruction to blood flow through the umbilical vessels, resulting in fetal morbidity and mortality. Edema, congestion, and thrombosis of the blood vessels may be present. Sections for histologic examination from the twisted area of the cord and its vicinity should be taken to assess the vascular changes.

Stricture of the Umbilical Cord

This lesion is characterized by a significant reduction in the diameter of a short segment of the umbilical cord in a macerated stillbirth at the fetal end (Figure 60). Strictured segment may also show torsion and marked constriction

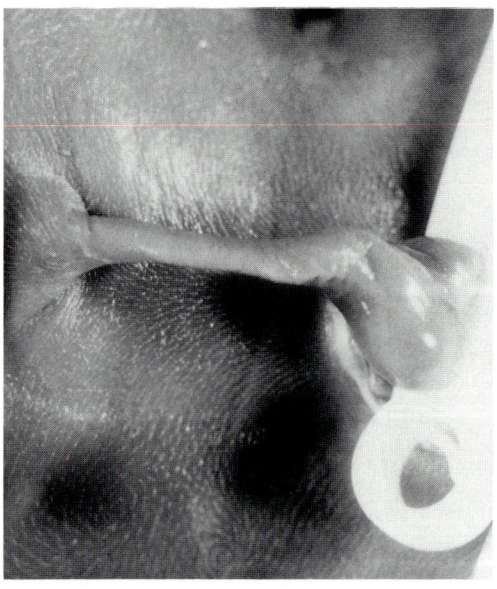

FIGURE 60. Stricture of the umbilical cord at the fetal end in a macerated stillborn. No torsion is present.

or luminal obliteration of the umbilical vessels. The umbilical vein distal to the stricture may show congestion or thrombosis. Primary segmental deficiency of Wharton's jelly has been considered as the cause of cord stricture (Figure 61). The umbilical cord should be carefully assessed grossly and histologically for these changes in the blood vessels and Wharton's jelly. There is some disagreement regarding the clinical significance of stricture. Stricture of the cord has been considered as the main cause of intrauterine death by some investigators. Others have considered it as a sequela of maceration starting at the fetal end of the cord in a fetus who died in utero due to other causes.[4,76,81,82] I have seen six cases of umbilical cord stricture, all associated with antepartum stillbirth with advanced maceration. The vascular changes of constriction in the strictured segment, as well as dilatation and congestion of umbilical vein distal to the stricture, were seen in only one of these six cases. Torsion of the cord was seen in another case. I consider stricture to be significant only when the vascular changes in the cord mentioned above are present.

Edema of the Umbilical Cord

Edema may be segmental (with pseudocyst formation) or diffuse. Focal edema may be seen around hematomas and in association with funisitis. The edematous cord has a swollen, pale, translucent appearance on the external and cut surfaces. In rare instances, the cord may be enlarged to as much as 5 cm in diameter. Coulter et al.[83] found 10% incidence of cord edema in all deliveries. It is more frequent in prematurity, cesarean delivery, abruptio placentae, diabetes, erythroblastosis fetalis, and intrauterine fetal death. DeSa[76] considers cord edema as a nonspecific change. Coulter et al.[83] found that cord edema was associated with idiopathic respiratory distress syndrome and transient tachypnea in the newborn but not with fetal distress. Increased hydrostatic and lower osmotic fetal intravascular pressures and increased water content of the fetus and placenta are considered as the predisposing factors for cord edema.[83]

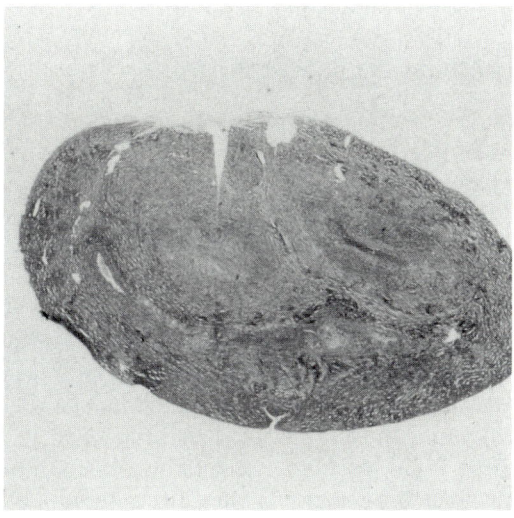

FIGURE 61. Strictured segment showing constriction of the umbilical vessels and lack of Wharton's jelly (H&E, ×12).

Embryonic Remnants of the Umbilical Cord

Four types of remnants are detected on histologic examination:

1. Vitellointestinal (omphalomesenteric) duct remnants, consisting of tubular structures (<1 mm in diameter), lined by cuboidal or columnar epithelium. Mucin-secreting cells are often present. Muscle coat may be seen around the epithelial lining.
2. Allantoic duct remnants, consisting of clusters of epithelial cells or microcystic structures lined by flattened epithelium.
3. Vascular remnants, consisting of thin-walled, capillary-like blood vessels. Cystic dilatation may occur in the first two types of remnants (see below). A microscopic focus of angioma-like proliferation of the vascular remnants may be present. The overall incidence of all three types of remnants is 23.1% in consecutive placentas.[84] No perinatal complications or congenital anomalies are usually found in association with these remnants.[84] However, in rare instances, the omphalomesenteric duct remnant may be lined by gastric epithelium containing acid-secreting cells. Ulceration of the duct remnant with intraamniotic hemorrhage resulting in fetal death has been described in one such case.[85]
4. Urachal remnants, occurring in association with the extremely rare malformation of persistent urachus, consisting of small cystic structures lined by transitional epithelium. The umbilical cord is turgid and swollen at birth. Urine drains from the umbilicus after the umbilical cord stump falls off.

Cysts of the Umbilical Cord

Cystic lesions may represent (1) true epithelium-lined cysts, (2) pseudocysts due to segmental edema or degeneration of Wharton's jelly, (3) neoplastic cysts (see below). The true cysts arise from allantoic and vitellointestinal duct remnants and from inclusions of amniotic epithelium. The cysts are small and have no clinical significance. However, in rare instances, a large cyst may compress the umbilical blood vessels. Large cysts can be visualized by ultrasound examination.

Tumors of the Umbilical Cord

There are two types of tumors: (1) hemangiomas and (2) teratomas. Both tumors are rare, but the former are relatively more common. Hemangiomas vary in size from 0.5 to 17 cm.[76,86] The associated cord edema and/or hematoma are often included in these measurements. Both capillary and cavernous types have been described. Sclerosis, myxomatous change, calcification, and osseous metaplasia can occur in the stroma of the hemangiomas. Arteriovenous fistulas and angiomatoid foci have also been described.[76] The hemangiomas arise from the umbilical blood vessels or persistent vascular remnants. Perinatal complications, hydramnios, or hemangiomas of the skin or viscera of the fetus are not usually associated with cord hemangiomas. However, large hemangiomas may be associated with IUGR, hydramnios and premature delivery.[4] Cord teratomas which are partly cystic and partly solid are benign tumors. As explained in the section in teratomas of the placenta, the germ cells may show aberrant migration into the cord.[4]

Prolapse of the Umbilical Cord

Long cords predispose to prolapse. In small premature infants the cord may prolapse through the space left between the improperly engaged presenting fetal part and the pelvic inlet. Prolapse is also more frequently seen in multiparous women, fetal malpresentation and premature onset of labor and following obstetric interventions including amniotomy.[86a] The prolapsed cord can get compressed with interference of the blood flow through the umbilical blood vessels. Thrombosis of the umbilical blood vessels, particularly the umbilical vein may rarely occur. Prolapse of umbilical cord is a clinical and not a pathologic diagnosis. It is associated with increased perinatal morbidity and mortality.

Entanglement of the Umbilical Cord

Entanglement may occur: a) in a twin placenta between two cords of a monochorionic monoamniotic twin placenta or b) in a singleton placenta with an abnormally long cord. The entanglement may involve wrapping of the cord around fetal parts such as neck (nuchal cord). Marks of the wrapped cord may be present on the involved fetal part. Tightly wrapped umbilical cord results in fetal asphyxia due to compression of the umbilical blood vessels. Increased traction on the cord forming loops around fetal parts may also occur.

Umbilical Vasculitis and Funisitis

These lesions are described in the section on chorioamnionitis.

LESIONS OF THE MEMBRANES

The amnion and chorion are passively attached to each other due to the internal pressure of the amniotic fluid. The two membranes can be readily separated from each in the gross specimen (Figure 62). The space between the two membranes, which is normally sterile, is the best site for taking cultures for pathogenic microorganisms. Histologically, the following layers can be recognized in the membranes: amnion composed of epithelial lining; basal lamina and mesoderm: an intermediate zone of loose collagen bundles and fibroblasts; and chorion composed of mesoderm, extravillous trophoblast, and atrophic villi (Figure 13). Decidua (fused decidua capsularis and decidua parietalis from 17 weeks of gestation) is attached to the chorion. Small amounts of fibrin are also present. The amniotic epithelium, which plays a role in the homeostasis of amniotic fluid, is of the columnar, cuboidal, or squamoid type. These differences may be artifacts of fixation and processing. The amnion is avascular. Fetal blood vessels extending from the chorionic plate are present in the chorion up to the sixth month of gestation. These vessels are absent in the chorion during the last trimester. The decidua attached to the membranes contains the maternal blood vessels, which show pathologic changes in maternal disorders such as hypertension and preeclampsia.

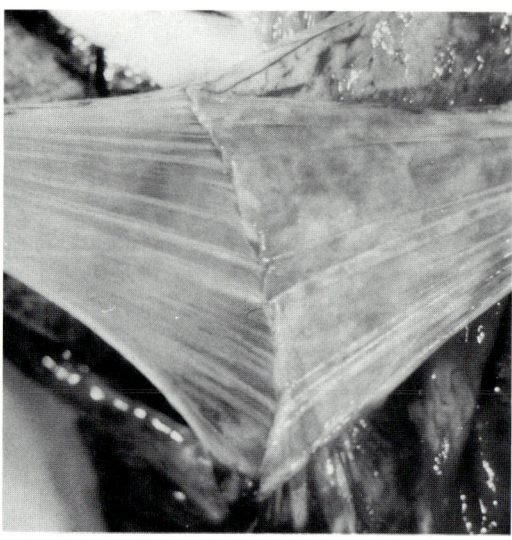

FIGURE 62. Amnion (on the left) can be easily separated from chorion by holding each in a forceps. A swab is placed in the space to take material for cultures.

Squamous Metaplasia

On gross examination, squamous metaplasia consists of gray or white plaques or slightly elevated foci measuring a few millimeters in diameter. There may be multiple lesions that tend to be concentrated around the cord insertion. The lesions, which are seen in about 25% of term placentas, are difficult to separate from the amnion. Histologically, keratinizing squamous epithelium is seen. The lesion has no clinical or pathologic significance.

Amnion Nodosum

In this condition, multiple small (1–5 mm), slightly raised, yellowish-white, readily detachable nodules are seen, particularly near the cord insertion on the fetal surface of the placenta (Figure 63). Lesions are also present on the extraplacental amnion and on the umbilical cord. The nodules are composed of amorphous and fibrillar eosinophilic material, squamous epithelial cells, and hair and are mixed with fatty sebaceous material (Figure 64). There is no inflammatory reaction. Therefore the term "vernix granuloma" is inappropriate. There may be intact amniotic epithelium underneath the nodules. Alternatively, amniotic epithelium may grow over the nodules. Landing,[87] who coined the term "amnion nodosum," was the first to recognize the association of amnion nodosum with oligohydramnios. It has been suggested that the cellular and noncellular debris is concentrated in the reduced amount of amniotic fluid seen in oligohydramnios and subsequently is compressed on the amniotic surface. Because of oligohydramnios, the amniotic epithelium may also be defective and "sticky." The clinical significance of amnion nodosum is that it is indicative of oligohydramnios and should alert the clinician to renal and/or urinary tract anomalies in the fetus (which cause oligohydramnios due to deficient or absent urinary output).

Lesions of the Membranes

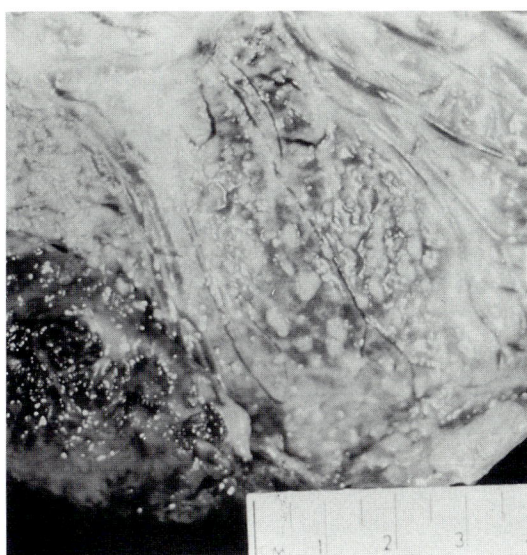

FIGURE 63. Whitish, slightly raised plaques of amnion nodosum on the membranes covering the fetal surface of the placenta.

Amniotic Cysts, Rests, and Polyps

These are rare. Cysts may arise from (1) localized edema (pseudocysts), (2) amniotic epithelial inclusions, or (3) rests of squamous epithelium underneath the epithelium. Cartilaginous and bony rests also occur. Amniotic polyps are composed of hyperplastic epithelium. Their significance is not known.

Amniotic Web

An amniotic web (also called "chorda") extends from the fetal surface of the placenta to the umbilical cord. It may restrict cord movement and may possibly interfere with circulation in the cord.[77] It is considered a developmental anomaly.

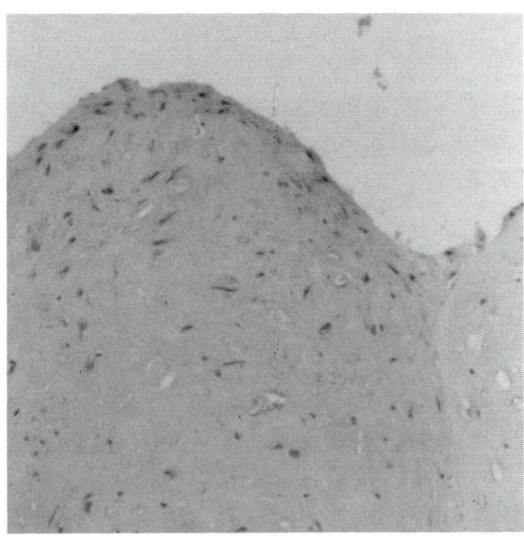

FIGURE 64. Amnion nodosum composed of eosinophilic, amorphous material with squames and vacuoles of fatty sebaceous material; there is no inflammatory reaction (H&E, ×100).

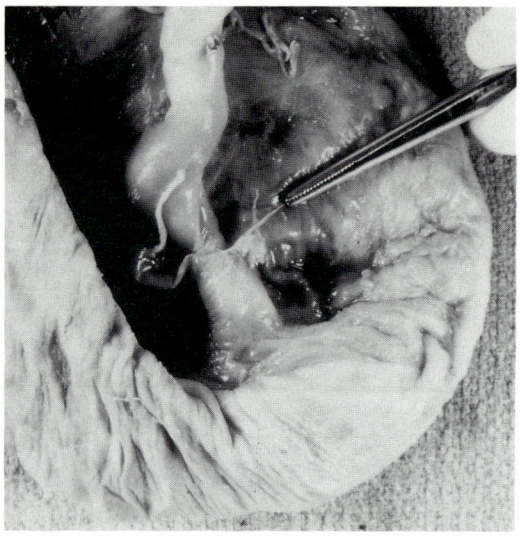

FIGURE 65. Note amniotic bands, one of which surrounds the umbilical cord in amniotic band syndrome.

Amniotic Band Syndrome (ABS)

ABS is characterized by the formation of amniotic bands in which fetal parts, including umbilical cord, become entangled (Figures 65, 66). The attachment between amnion and chorion is said to be fully developed at 12 weeks of gestation. However, according to sonographic findings, the attachment is fully developed at 17 weeks. Therefore, it is assumed that rupture of amnion, with its detachment from the chorion, can occur before 12–17 weeks of gestation. The detached amnion becomes fragmented and rolled up to form band(s)[88] that may encircle the umbilical cord, resulting in its strangulation and intrauterine death.[89] Fetal parts may also get entangled in these bands. The amniotic fluid is

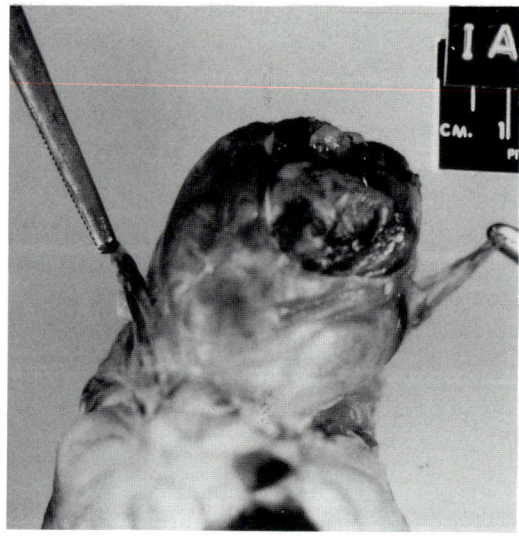

FIGURE 66. Amniotic bands held by forceps producing constricting grooves of the head with severe malformation of the cranial bones and the brain.

absorbed by the chorion, and the resulting oligohydramnios produces club feet. The amniotic bands adhere to the areas of skin abrasion and may be swallowed by the fetus, resulting in facial clefts. Compression of fetal parts results from loss of the cushioning effect of amniotic fluid. The following categories of anomalies are recognized: (1) *limb anomalies*—constriction rings, amputation, fenestrated syndactyly, club feet; (2) *craniofacial anomalies*—facial and cranial clefting, encephalocele, excencephaly, cleft lip, cleft palate, microphthalmia, nasal defects; (3) *parietal anomalies*—gastroschisis, thoracic wall defects; (4) *umbilical cord anomalies*—strangulation. In some cases, multiple amniotic bands surround various fetal parts, producing multiple anomalies, amputations, thoracic and abdominal wall defects, and a grossly malformed fetus. Spontaneous abortion may occur or the patient may agree to have the pregnancy terminated. In such cases, both the placenta and the fetus will be submitted to the surgical pathologist. The placenta in ABS shows tearing apart of the amnion from the chorion. Remnants of amnion can be found in the form of amniotic bands or strings (Figure 65). The latter may be delicate and may be missed. In such cases, the placenta should be examined carefully under water.

The cause of rupture of the amnion remains uncertain. Trauma during pregnancy and hereditary collagen defects occurring in metabolic disorders such as osteogenesis imperfecta or Ehlers–Danlos syndrome (characterized by abnormalities of collagen, fibronectin, etc.) have been implicated.[5,90] There are few well-documented cases of ABS following maternal trauma.[88] Most investigators consider amniotic rupture, presumably a spontaneous event, as the basic abnormality in ABS and the fetal anomalies a consequence of disruption by the amniotic bands. This view has been challenged by Lockwood et al.,[91] who have suggested that ABS is a consequence of epiblastic damage to both the amnion and the embryo, and is a result of a multifactorial process resulting in malformations and disruptions. ABS has also been called "early amnion rupture sequence." It does not usually recur in subsequent pregnancies.

Features such as asymmetry of missing parts, constricting grooves on the skin, with edema distally, fenestrated syndactyly, and demonstration of amniotic bands attached to or encircling fetal parts enable the diagnosis of ABS. The amniotic nature of the bands should be confirmed by histologic examination showing connective tissue lined by amniotic epithelium (Figure 67). There are no inflammatory or degenerative changes.

Apparent amniotic bands may be seen on ultrasonography in some pregnancies without detectable amniotic bands on placental examination at delivery. This potential pitfall in the sonographic diagnosis may result from the presence of decidual bands adherent to previously damaged endometrium (previous abortion, myomectomy, infection, etc.). More detailed studies are necessary to elucidate the precise nature of this condition.[5,92]

Extramembranous Pregnancy

Both amnion and chorion may rupture during pregnancy, with intermittent leakage of amniotic fluid and development of the fetus outside the membranous sac. The placenta in such extramembranous pregnancy is always circumvallate and has a small, membranous sac. It has been suggested that the small size of the

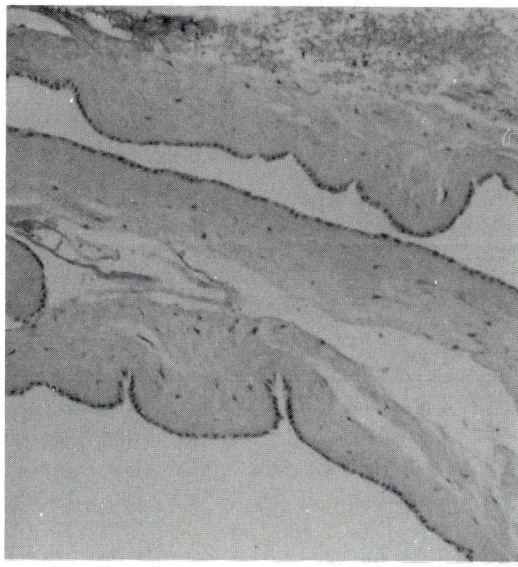

FIGURE 67. Histologic section of one of the bands from Figure 66 confirms that it is composed of amnion (H&E, ×100).

membranous sac in such a placenta makes it more prone to rupture as a result of stretching induced by fetal growth. It is also conceivable that the membranes may rupture due to trauma. Premature delivery usually occurs in extramembranous pregnancy.

Extraamniotic Pregnancy

The amnion alone may rupture, without formation of bands. Fetal development occurs inside the intact chorion. The placenta shows a thickened remnant of amnion, usually around the umbilical cord. No amniotic bands are seen in this condition.

Meconium Staining of the Membranes

Meconium staining of membranes occurs when the fetus passes meconium in the amniotic fluid. The obstetrician recognizes the meconium as yellow-green material in the dispersed foam or as thick lumps in the amniotic fluid, or observes meconium covering the perineum or other parts of the fetus. The obstetrician should record these findings on the surgical pathology form so that the pathologist is alerted to look for evidence of meconium staining on gross and microscopic examination of the extraplacental membranes and the membranes covering the fetal surface of the placenta.

Significance of Meconium

Meconium is not usually passed before 30 weeks of gestation since the level of motilin, the hormone related to intestinal motor activity, is low in premature infants.[5] However, a rare case of passage and aspiration of meconium has been reported at 27 weeks' gestation.[93] Traditionally, passing of meconium is considered a response to fetal distress. However, meconium may be passed in the absence of fetal distress, and not all fetuses with distress all pass meconium. Our understanding of the significance of meconium passage is still incomplete.[94,95]

Time Interval between Meconium Passage and Birth

Meconium staining of amniotic fluid is more common than that of membranes (19% vs. 10%).[96,97] The exact length of time which grossly demonstrable meconium staining of membranes takes is not known. Fujikura and Klionsky[97] state that it takes a minimum of 4–6 hours. Miller et al.[98] demonstrated minimal and maximal staining on gross examination after 1 hour and 3 to 6 hours of exposure, respectively, in in vitro experiments (immersion of membranes and umbilical cord in saline containing various concentrations of meconium at various temperatures). In these experiments, macrophages containing brown granular pigment were seen histologically in the amnion and chorion after 1- and 3-hour exposures, respectively. These figures cannot be extrapolated to the in vivo clinical situation since the concentration of meconium and the rate of response may vary in individual patients.[99] It should also be noted that meconium may be passed more than once, and that meconium may travel through the amnion and even the chorion in a placenta after delivery if it is not refrigerated or not fixed in formalin.

Pathologic Features of Meconium Staining

The amniotic side of the free membranes and those covering the fetal surface are stained greenish to green on gross examination. The yellowish-green exudate present in severe chorioamnionitis may be mistaken for meconium staining on gross examination. On microscopic examination, one or more of the following features are present: (1) amniotic debris sticking to the amniotic surface, showing yellow or yellow-brown discoloration (Figure 68) or (2) macrophages containing brown granular pigment in the cytoplasm or diffuse brown staining of the cytoplasm are present in the amnion and/or chorion (Figures 69, 70). The

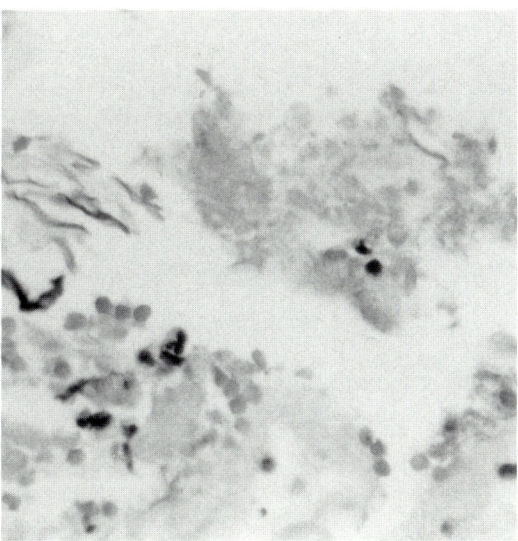

FIGURE 68. Brownish granular pigment lying free and/or staining the amniotic debris in meconium staining of the membranes (H&E, ×100).

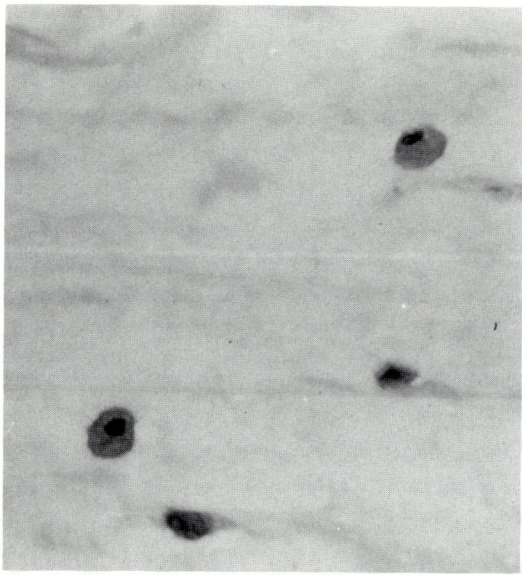

FIGURE 69. Macrophages in the amnion showing diffuse brown staining of the cytoplasm in meconium staining of the membranes (H&E, ×400).

pigment is negative for Perl's reaction for iron. In doubtful cases, Perl's reaction should be done since hemosiderin may be present occasionally in the membranes. Hemosiderin can also be distinguished from meconium pigment by the refractile, coarse, granular appearance of the former. A diagnosis of meconium-containing macrophage(s) should be made only when convincing brown pigment or diffuse brown staining of the cytoplasm is present. The macrophages may also show vacuolation of the cytoplasm (Figure 69). Occasionally there may be only rare to occasional macrophages in the membranes. A diligent and careful search of the sections of rolls of membranes and the fetal surface of the placenta

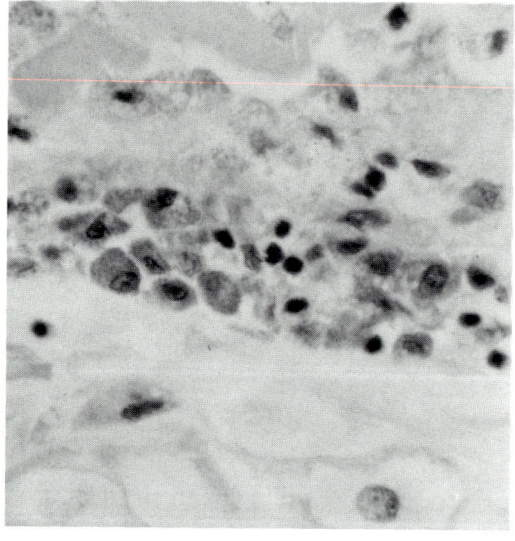

FIGURE 70. Macrophages in the chorion showing brown granular pigment in the cytoplasm in meconium staining of the membranes; the cytoplasm of the macrophages is vacuolated or evenly stained (H&E, ×400).

is essential before ruling out the presence of such macrophages. Mucicarmine stain and immunoperoxidase stain for carcinoembryonic antigen may light up these macrophages. However, in my experience with a diligent search and stringent criteria, the diagnosis of meconium-containing macrophages can be made on routine H&E stain. In some cases in which meconium staining is present on gross examination, a number of macrophages without any demonstrable pigment may be seen in the amnion (Figure 71). In rare instances, meconium-containing macrophages may be found in the membranes in the absence of appreciable greenish discoloration of the membranes on gross examination.

Other findings related to meconium staining are degeneration, vacuolation, necrosis, and stratification of the amniotic epithelium. Altshuler and Hyde[100] described meconium pigment-containing macrophages in Wharton's jelly and necrosis of muscle coat of the umbilical and placental blood vessels. They suggested that meconium may cause hypoperfusion of the fetus due to vasoconstriction of the umbilical blood vessels.

Acute Chorioamnionitis (ACA)

Definition

ACA can be defined in histologic, clinical, and microbiologic terms. Histologically, it is characterized by an acute inflammatory infiltrate in one or more of the following structures: the extraplacental membrane, chorionic plate and its undersurface, or blood vessels in the chorionic plate and umbilical cord.[101] Inflammatory changes may be absent in individual sections of one or more of these structures. Therefore, sections from all of these structures should be routinely assessed for evidence of ACA. The inflammatory changes are more consistently found in the sections that include the site of rupture of the membranes and the undersurface of the chorionic plate.[101,102] Clinically, ACA is characterized by fever (≤38°C), leukocytosis, uterine tenderness in the mother,

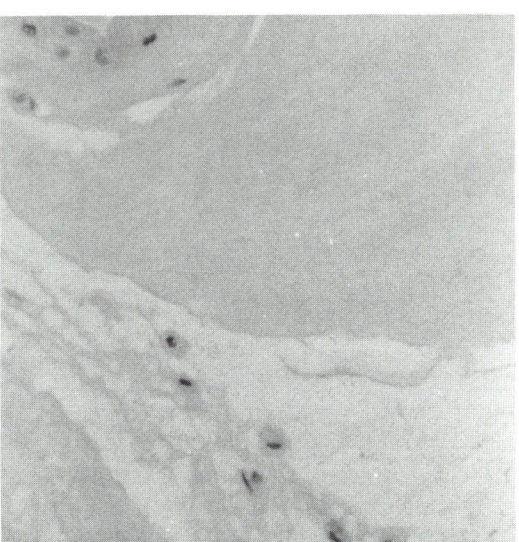

FIGURE 71. Numerous macrophages are present in the amnion. None of them contain brown pigment or show brown staining of the cytoplasm (H&E, ×250).

and turbid or foul-smelling amniotic fluid. In many cases, only fever may be present. The other features are present only in severe cases. In those cases in which no maternal signs are present and ACA is diagnosed histologically, the lesion is considered "silent" ACA. In group B streptococcal (GBS) infection, cultures from the maternal genital tract and the neonate may be positive in the absence of demonstrable chorioamnionitis.[102] Such cases may be considered as ACA in microbiologic terms.

Etiology

Various organisms present in the maternal genital tract—such as GBS, *Escherichia coli*, staphylococci, pseudomonas, proteus, and klebsiella—are among the common causes of ACA. Anaerobic organisms (*Clostridium perfringens, C. fusobacterium*) and particularly mycoplasma (*Ureaplasma urealyticum*) have also been recognized as important causes of ACA. *Chlamydia trachomatis*, which causes acute cervicitis, has been implicated as a cause of premature rupture of membranes and chorioamnionitis. A rat model of chlamydial chorioamnionitis has been described. However, there is no definitive evidence that chlamydia causes chorioamnionitis in humans, and it has not been isolated from the placenta. Among the fungi, candida is the most important organism. Viruses rarely produce ACA (see the section on specific viral villitis).

For the diagnosis of the etiologic agent, cultures should be taken from the material collected by swabs placed in the space between the chorion and amnion after peeling off the amnion from the chorion (Figure 62). The material for culture is best collected in the delivery room. Anaerobic culture and culture for mycoplasma should be set up. If these guidelines are not followed, negative cultures may be obtained in 50% of the cases. Because of the negative results on routinely processed cultures and lack of clinical manifestations in the mother and fetus in such a high proportion of cases with histologic ACA, some investigators have suggested that noninfectious factors such as the maternal immunological reaction to fetal tissue, gastric juice, amniotic debris, meconium, and pH changes in and hypertonicity of the amniotic fluid may be the cause(s) of ACA. Lauweryns et al.[103] failed to produce any inflammatory reaction in the membranes (or fetal lungs) when amniotic debris, meconium, gastric juice, and acidified amniotic fluid were injected into the amniotic sac of pregnant rabbits. They concluded that ACA is always infectious in origin. Further, as indicated above, the high proportion of negative results of culture are related to a lack of proper methods, and the absence of clinical manifestations may be due to low virulence of the infecting organisms.

The route of infection is via the maternal genital tract or, rarely, via acute villitis secondary to hematogenous spread. The most important predisposing factors to ACA are incompetent cervix, increased uterine activity (associated, e.g., with orgasm), instrumentation and vaginal examination. Since the membranes at the cervical os are exposed first to the infecting organisms, the inflammatory infiltration on microscopic examination is most severe at the site of the rupture of membranes (which should be at the center of the section of the roll of membranes taken for histologic examination). It should be noted that the membranes of most placentas at the site of rupture show a mild neutrophilic infiltrate unrelated to ACA. Such an infiltrate is apparently related to trauma to

FIGURE 72. (A) Acute chorioamnionitis characterized by moderately severe neutrophilic infiltration of the chorion, with extension of the amnion (H&E, ×100). (B) Acute chorioamnionitis with acute inflammatory infiltration in the undersurface of the chorionic plate (H&E, ×100).

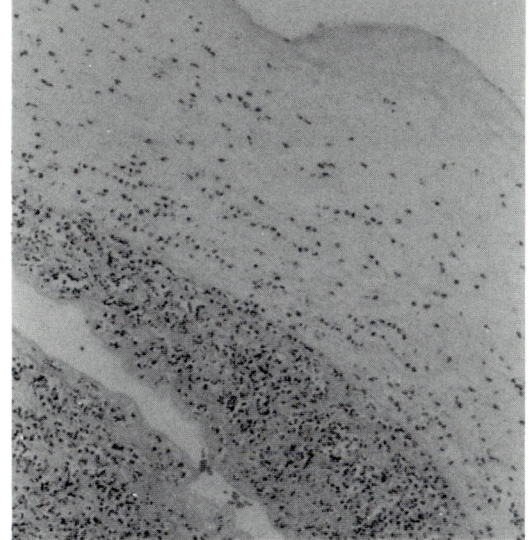

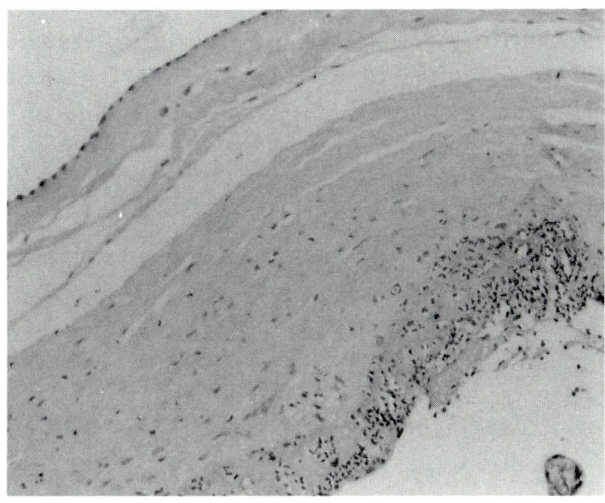

the membranes from the presenting fetal part. The neutrophilic response to the infection is from the maternal decidual blood vessels. Thus the inflammatory cells in the membranes are of maternal origin. The neutrophils first infiltrate the chorion, to which they may be confined in many cases. Variable extension to the amnion is seen in some cases (Figure 72, 73). In dichorionic diamniotic twin placenta, ACA may remain confined to twin A. ACA of twin B is never seen in the absence of ACA of twin A. The organisms and neutrophils also spread to the amniotic fluid and upward toward the chorionic plate. The umbilical cord is exposed to the organisms in the amniotic fluid, and there is a fetal neutrophilic response originating from the umbilical vein first and later from the arteries

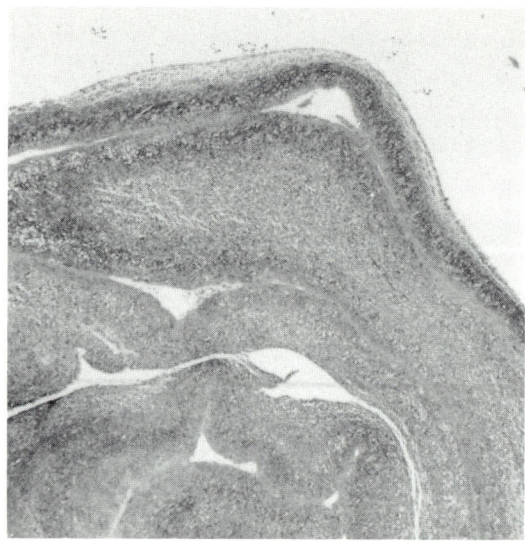

FIGURE 73. Severe diffuse neutrophilic infiltrate in both the chorion and amnion (H&E, ×40).

(umbilical vasculitis with funisitis). Umbilical vasculitis and funisitis are eccentric since the inflammatory response is directed toward the organisms in the amniotic cavity. Umbilical vasculitis does not extend beyond the abdominal wall of the fetus. ACA spreads to the undersurface of the chorionic plate. Maternal neutrophils originating from the intervillous space are seen at this site. A fetal neutrophilic response is seen in the chorion, amnion, and placental blood vessels of the chorionic plate. This vasculitis does not extend beyond the chorionic plate to the branches of the placental blood vessels or the villi. However, focal acute villitis may occur if there is fetal septicemia secondary to pulmonary aspiration of infected amniotic fluid and fetal pneumonia (Figure 74). The neutrophilic response in ACA may vary from minimal and focal to severe and diffuse. Occasional isolated neutrophils may be found in the membranes or at the undersurface of the chorionic plate. Only when moderate to large numbers of neutrophils are present, or when they are present in clusters of five or more, is a diagnosis of ACA indicated. As noted above, in GBS infection, for example, no inflammatory response may be present.[102] The nuclei of the cells of the chorion may show pyknosis (Figure 75), which may be mistaken for neutrophilic infiltration. It is important to emphasize that in occasional cases of ACA, a neutrophilic infiltrate may be seen only in the underface of the chorionic plate. In longstanding infection, a plasmacytic infiltrate may be found in the membranes and lungs, along with the neutrophilic infiltrate.[5]

Clinical Significance

As indicated above, the fetus may develop intrauterine pneumonia secondary to aspiration of infected amniotic fluid, followed by septicemia and intrauterine death or neonatal morbidity and mortality (Figure 74). This complication of ACA is seen infrequently, and the presence of ACA, with or without funisitis, does not necessarily mean that there is fetal sepsis. Infected amniotic fluid is also swallowed into the gastrointestinal tract and aspirated into the middle ears.[5,104]

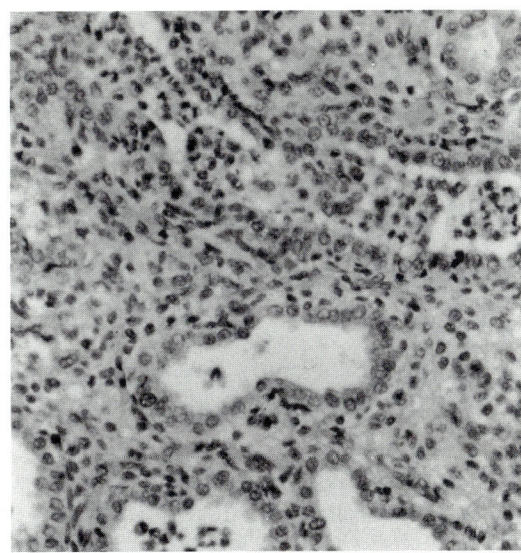

FIGURE 74. Intrauterine pneumonia characterized by a neutrophilic infiltrate in the alveoli and the alveolar septa (H&E, ×100).

Maternal sepsis also is infrequent. The most important and most frequent complication of ACA appears to be the initiation of premature labor. Phospholipases from the bacteria and neutrophils of ACA cause the release of prostaglandins from the membranes.[101] Uterine contractions and dilatation of the cervix due to prostaglandin release herald the onset of premature labor. Collagenases and elastases of neutrophilic origin produce rupture of the membranes. Premature labor culminates in delivery of a premature infant, with all the sequelae of prematurity in the newborn infant who, in addition, may have intrauterine pneumonia. ACA has been implicated as a cause in about one-third of the cases of preterm delivery. In a prospective, case-controlled study, Hillier et al.[105] have shown that infection of the chorioamnion is strongly related to histologic chorioamnionitis and may be related to premature birth. The organisms which

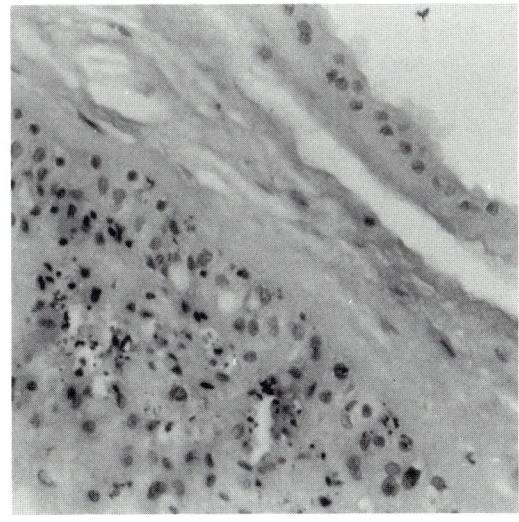

FIGURE 75. Nuclear pyknosis of cells of chorion, which should not be mistaken for neutrophilic infiltrate. (H&E, ×250).

were most frequently isolated included *Ureaplasma urealyticum* and *Gardnerella vaginalis*. Other investigators have implicated *C. trachomatis*, *N. gonorrheae*, *T. vaginalis*, GBS, *M. hominis* and *Bacteroides* species with prematurity.

Thus, it needs to be emphasized that although ACA is the *result of prolonged* rupture of membranes in some cases, it is the *cause of premature* rupture of membranes in other cases. Organisms can spread to the membranes in the absence of rupture of the amniotic sac, producing premature rupture of membranes and ACA. Loss or diminution of bactericidal factors (lysozyme, immunoglobulins etc) in the amniotic fluid due to prematurity, presence of meconium or unknown reasons may contribute to the occurrence of ACA.[106,107]

Chronic Chorioamnionitis (CCA)

CCA, which is rare, is characterized by infiltration of the free membranes by mature lymphocytes, with or without an admixture of variable numbers of plasma cells, histiocytes, immature lymphocytes and immunoblasts. The chorionic plate and blood vessels of the umbilical cord may also be involved.[108,109] In most cases of CCA, there is accompanying chronic necrotizing lymphohistiocytic villitis of varying degrees of severity. In most cases, the etiology of CCA is not known. However, occurrence of CCA in rare cases of HSV infection, syphilis and toxoplasmosis suggests that it may have an infectious etiology. Immunologic factors may be involved in some cases. The mothers showing CCA had various problems during the antenatal period, including hypertension, diabetes, isoimmunization, and disseminated intravascular coagulation. The preterm delivery of a low-birth-weight infant in 13 of the 17 cases reported by Gersell et al. may be related to concomitant chronic villitis.[108]

Funisitis

Funisitis is almost always associated with ACA. (Isolated funisitis may occur in the segment of the umbilical cord that prolapses or is compressed against the uterine wall. Eosinophils may be admixed or may be the only inflammatory cells in some cases of isolated funisitis. The cause and significance of presence of eosinophils in the inflammatory infiltrate are not known.) Besides the funisitis and umbilical vasculitis occurring as part of ACA, specific types of funisitis also occur. Necrotizing funisitis, characterized by whitish areas of necrosis around the umbilical vessels seen on the cut surface of the cord, has been described in syphilitic infection.[36] However, necrotizing funisitis is not diagnostic of congenital syphilis since in many cases the etiologic agent cannot be detected.[110] Pale yellow plaques are seen on the surface of the cord on gross examination in *Candida funisitis*.[111] Sclerosing funisitis is characterized by a rigid cord in which sclerosis and an inflammatory exudate are seen around the umbilical blood vessels. The etiology remains undetermined in many cases.

Amniotic Fluid Embolism (AME)

This can lead to the death of the mother. AME occurs during cesarean section, or in patients with placenta previa or agitated labor. Amniotic fluid appears to enter through large uteroplacental veins. Amniotic debris dissecting between the amnion and chorion can be demonstrated in some normal placentas; such a finding is not considered the initial event in AME. Diagnosis of AME is made by demonstrating vernix (desquamated epithelial cells) in maternal peripheral blood smears. In fatal cases, sections of the lungs show squames and hair in the branches of pulmonary arteries. Placental examination is not helpful in making the diagnosis.

Tumors of the Placental Membranes

Placental teratomas, described above, lie between the amnion and chorion on the fetal surface or at the placental margin. Therefore, these tumors can be considered to arise primarily in the membranes. A localized thickening in the membranes related to a vanishing twin may be mistaken for a tumor (see the section on twin pregnancy).

ABNORMALITIES OF THE DECIDUA

Terminology

(1) *Decidua basalis* (DB)—decidua at the maternal surface of the placental disk; (2) *decidua capsularis* (DC)—decidua attached to the membranes of the protruding embryo; (3) *decidua parietalis* (DP) (or *decidua vera*)—decidua lining the uterine cavity (Figure 1). DC fuses with the DP from 17 weeks' gestation since the membranes come into contact with the uterine wall, largely obliterating the uterine cavity.

Deciduitis

A few small foci of an acute inflammatory infiltrate are present in the decidua in most placentas. Fox considers this degree of inflammation almost physiological.[4] A pathologic diagnosis of deciduitis is not made in such instances. Large foci of a severe, acute inflammatory infiltrate and necrosis are essential for such a diagnosis. Acute deciduitis of this type is often accompanied by ACA. The mother may also show signs of local or generalized sepsis. Chronic deciduitis characterized by a lymphoplasmacytic infiltrate can occur in cases of specific villitis and VUE (Figure 76).

Decidual Vasculopathy

The maternal arteries present in the decidua show the vascular changes associated with preeclampsia and hypertension (see the sections on maternal vasculature, preeclampsia, and hypertension).

LESIONS OF THE PLACENTA IN MATERNAL DISORDERS (Table 7)

Toxemia of Pregnancy

Gross Features
The weight of the placenta is reduced or may be within normal limits. Infarcts involving >5% of the placenta are commonly seen. In severe preeclampsia, more than 50% of the placenta may show infarcts. Retroplacental hematoma may be present.

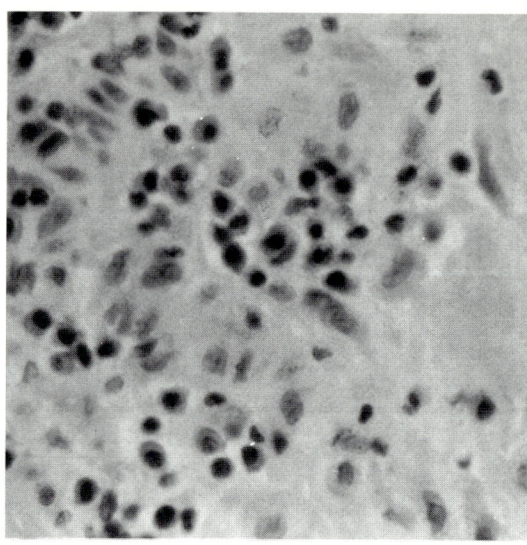

FIGURE 76. Lymphoplasmacytic infiltrate in the decidua (H&E, ×250).

Histologic Features

The villi may show accelerated maturation. There is reduced vascularity of the villi when fibromuscular hyperplasia and obliterative endarteritis of the fetal stem arteries are present. Edema, stromal fibrosis, prominent and increased numbers of syncytial knots, cytotrophoblastic hyperplasia, (cytotrophoblast in >20–40% of vili at term), trophoblastic basement membrane thickening (in >3% of villi), (Figure 27), deficiency of the vasculosyncytial membrane, and excessive fibrinoid necrosis may also be seen in the villi. As indicated above in the section on histologic abnormalities, PAS stain and thin sections of plastic embedded material enhance the recognition of cytotrophoblastic hyperplasia. In my experience, it is not a readily demonstrable finding in routine histologic sections. The basic and most consistent lesion is acute atherosis in the basal arteries in the decidua basalis and the spiral arteries in the decidua parietalis, characterized by fibrinoid necrosis and lipid macrophages in the vessel wall and the perivascular lymphocytic infiltration (see the section on maternal vasculature) (Figures 40, 41). Occlusive thrombosis may be seen in the arteries affected by acute atherosis, particularly when infarcts are present. Careful examination of these arteries in the decidua attached to the membrane rolls and along the maternal surface is essential to recognize this lesion. Extra sections from these sites may be taken to enhance the probability of having an adequate sample of maternal arteries for histologic assessment.

Pathogenesis

The lesions in the villi are direct sequelae of ischemia due to what is considered inadequate placentation in early pregnancy. In preeclampsia there is inadequate physiologic transformation of intramyometrial portions of spiral arteries due to failure of trophoblastic infiltration, so that narrow, undilated segments between the radial arteries and the decidual portions of the spiral artery persist throughout pregnancy (see the section on maternal uteroplacental blood vessels and Figure 39). This ischemia is further compounded by acute atherosis of the uteroplacental maternal arteries. Infarcts are related to occlusive thrombi in the maternal arteries and arterioles and to the retroplacental hematoma. Retroplacental hematoma is due to rupture of arteries affected by acute atherosis. Cytotrophoblastic hyperplasia and thickening of the trophoblastic basement membrane are manifestations of uteroplacental ischemia. The pathogenesis of the basic lesion (i.e., acute atherosis) is not known. There is accumulation of lipid in muscle cells in the arteries. Necrosis of these cells results in release of the lipid, which is phagocytosed by the macrophages. An immunopathologic basis has been implicated since there is deposition of IgM, fibrinoid and C3 in the involved arteries.

Comment

In some cases, particularly those with mild toxemia, the placenta may not show any recognizable gross and microscopic lesions. This may be partly due to the absence of maternal arteries in the sections (including the extra ones) taken for histologic assessment. The most characteristic primary histologic lesion is acute atherosis of maternal arteries. A granulomatous reaction around decidual arteries may be seen on rare occasions.[5] Prominent and excessive numbers of syncytial knots (Tenney–Parker change) have been emphasized as a characteristic finding.[5] Tenney–Parker change is more readily recognizable in a premature or preterm placenta. Although some investigators claim to have observed acute atherosis in hypertension, systemic lupus erythematosus (SLE), diabetes and IUGR,[112,113] it appears that from a practical point of view, acute atherosis can be considered diagnostic of toxemia of pregnancy. The other histologic features, such as cytotrophoblastic hyperplasia and trophoblastic basement membrane thickening, are difficult to demonstrate consistently.

If maternal arteries are present in the decidua, acute atherosis is readily recognizable. In my experience, sections from the margin of the placenta, along with the attached membranes, tend to show maternal arteries more frequently than sections from the maternal surface. However, in some cases, the absence of maternal arteries or of an adequate amount of decidua, even in the additional sections of the placenta and membranes, makes assessment of maternal vascular changes associated with preeclampsia impossible. A comment to that effect should be added in the surgical pathology report. In occasional cases diagnosed clinically as preeclampsia, no maternal vascular lesions may be seen. It is possible that the clinical diagnosis may have been inappropriate. Conversely, acute atherosis may be seen rarely in the absence of overt clinical features of preeclampsia. It is possible that in such cases the disease process of preeclampsia is present in the subclinical form.

In the HELLP syndrome, characterized by hemolysis, elevated liver enzymes, and low platelets, which is more commonly seen in white women,[114] the placental pathologic lesions are similar to those in preeclampsia. (The HELLP syndrome is considered an extremely severe variant of preeclampsia.) The lesions may be more severe, and the incidence of thrombosis of maternal arteries may be more frequent. A systematic description of placental findings in the HELLP syndrome is lacking in the literature.

Maternal Hypertension

The placenta shows the same findings as those described above for preeclampsia, with three exceptions: (1) the maternal vasculature in the decidua shows medial thickening and intimal hyperplasia (Figure 42)—acute atherosis is seldom seen in essential hypertension (see above), (2) there is no excess of fibrinoid necrosis of villi, and (3) the frequency and severity of obliterative endarteritis of stem villi are less marked than in preeclampsia (therefore, the prominence of syncytial knots and stromal fibrosis of villi is also less marked).[4]

Maternal Diabetes

Gross Features

Increased weight, pallor and a high incidence (~10%) of single umbilical artery have been described (see the criteria for the diagnosis of large placenta above). In addition to a generalized pale appearance, localized, well-demarcated areas of increased pallor due to fetal artery thrombosis may be present.

Histologic Features

Edema, variable maturity (normal in 40%, delayed or accelerated in 30% each), stromal fibrosis, prominent syncytial knots (or increased syncytial sprouting) and cytotrophoblast, thickening of the trophoblastic basement membrane, variable vascularity (normal, hypovascularity or chorangiosis), and excessive fibrinoid necrosis of villi have been described. The fetal stem arteries show thrombosis in about 10% of cases (4.5% of normal placentas show this finding). Obliterative endarteritis is also seen in 25% of cases (normally, 10% of placentas show this finding). Endothelial swelling and syncytial necrosis are seen by electron microscopy. No lesions are present in the decidual maternal arteries unless diabetes is complicated by preexisting hypertension or superimposed preeclampsia (see above).

Pathogenesis

The pathogenesis of these lesions is not clear. The excessive number of cytotrophoblasts may be an expression of failure of regression because of delayed maturation of villi. Since there is no narrowing of maternal arteries in uncomplicated diabetes, ischemia cannot explain the pathogenesis of the lesions. Immunologic factors such as immune complexes of insulin and antiinsulin antibodies have been implicated in the pathogenesis of fibrinoid necrosis of villi, trophoblastic basement membrane thickening, and obliterative endarteritis of fetal stem arteries. An abnormal internal metabolic environment in a diabetic mother may also be related to the pathogenesis.

Comment

There are no specific or consistent placental abnormalities in maternal diabetes. The placenta may be normal in many cases. Correlation between the severity and duration of diabetes (Table 8) and the severity of placental lesions has not been established. Detailed morphometric comparison of histologic and electron microscopic features seen in placentas of diabetic and nondiabetic normal women has revealed few statistically significant differences.[115,116]

TABLE 7 Salient Features of the Placenta in Maternal Disorders

Disorders	Salient gross features	Salient microscopic features	Comment
Toxemia of pregnancy	Low weight, infarcts (>5%), retroplacental hematoma	Villi—accelerated maturation, prominent cytotrophoblastic hyperplasia, thickening of trophoblastic basement membrane; maternal arteries—acute atherosis (fibrinoid necrosis, lipid macrophages); thrombosis of vessels may be present	Placenta may be normal in mild cases; severe lesions tend to occur in severe cases; additional sections from the membranes and maternal surface of the placenta may be needed to get adequate sample of maternal arteries; HELLP syndrome shows similar but more severe lesions
Maternal hypertension	Low weight, infarcts (>5%), retroplacental hematoma	Villi—same as in toxemia, except for less prominence of syncytial knots; maternal arteries—intimal hyperplasia and medial thickening	Toxemia of pregnancy may be superimposed on hypertension
Maternal diabetes	Increased weight, generalized pallor, high incidence of single umbilical artery, localized pallor due to fetal artery thrombosis	Villi—edema, variable maturity (normal, delayed, or accelerated) and vascularity, obliterative endarteritis, thrombosis of fetal stem arteries	Maternal vascular lesions are not seen in diabetes without hypertension or toxemia of pregnancy; the placenta may be normal; lesions are less severe and less frequent in gestational diabetes
Abortion	Torsion, stricture and true knot of the cord, massive subchorial thrombosis, partial hydatidiform mole, maternal floor infarction	Villi: (1) normal or (2) stromal fibrosis with prominent trophoblast or (3) hydropic change with hypo- or avascularity of villi or (4) hydatidiform change when partial mole or (5) hypoplastic villi	In hydropic change, there is no circumferential trophoblastic hyperplasia; DNA analysis of the placental tissue by flow cytometry and/or image cytometry should be done if hydatidiform change is present

TABLE 7 (Continued)

Disorders	Salient gross features	Salient microscopic features	Comment
Premature labor and delivery	Placental findings related to associated obstetrical or maternal condition such as abruptio placentae, preeclampsia, hypertension, diabetes, chorioamnionitis	Placental findings in otherwise normal pregnancies: variable villous maturation (delayed, accelerated, or normal for the gestational age), higher incidence of fibrinoid necrosis of villi	In many cases, there is no detectable associated condition; the placenta may be normal for the gestational age
Postmaturity	Heavy placenta, infarct, and calcification (not more frequent than in term placentas)	Villi: stromal fibrosis, prominent trophoblast, thickened trophoblastic basement membrane, obliterative endarteritis of fetal stem arteries, variable vascularity (normal, hypovascular)	Some cases may be misdiagnosed due to incorrect calculation of the gestational age
Polyhydramnios (>2000 ml)	Seen in association with fetal malformations (e.g., esophageal atresia), twin transfusion syndrome, maternal diabetes, and chorioangioma	No histologic changes related to polyhydroamnios	Placental findings are related to the maternal or fetal condition present in the particular case (e.g., vascular anastomoses in twin transfusion syndrome)
Oligohydramnios	Seen in postmaturity, fetal urinary tract obstruction, and renal anomalies (e.g., renal agenesis), chronic leakage of amniotic fluid; amnion nodosum is the characteristic lesion	Amnion nodosum	Chorionamnionitis is present with chronic leakage of amniotic fluid
Premature, preterm, and prolonged rupture of membranes	Retroplacental hematoma tends to occur more frequently in patients with premature rupture of membranes	Acute chorionamnionitis	Cultures should be taken in the delivery room in all of these cases; see the section on chorioamnionitis for details

Maternal fever		Malarial parasites may be present in the intervillous space in cases of maternal malaria; placenta may not show any lesion in some cases of maternal fever
Maternal substance abuse	Low weight, retroplacental hematoma, premature rupture of membranes, and meconium staining are seen with higher frequency in different types of substance abuse	Placenta may be normal; see text for details of lesions seen in individual forms of substance abuse (alcohol, tobacco, cocaine, and heroin)
Abruptio placentae	Retroplacental hematoma with/without infarction of the overlying placental territory	Retroplacental hematoma is present in only 30% of cases of abruptio placentae; the blood clot may become detached and may not be sent with the specimen or it may be lost as vaginal bleeding; depression on the maternal surface, with or without an accompanying blood clot, can be considered evidence of retroplacental hematoma
Systemic lupus erythematosus (SLE)	Infarct (>25%), retroplacental hematoma	Acute atherosis with thrombosis can also occur in women with lupus anticoagulant in the absence of SLE; preeclampsia may be superimposed on SLE; therefore, the vascular lesions probably reflect the former

Note: rows for "Maternal fever" middle column and similar: Chorioamnionitis, villitis, and funistis related to specific viruses, bacteria, fungi or parasites are the main lesions seen in the placenta; Chorioamnionitis, villitis, hypovascularity of villi, and stromal fibrosis; Lesions associated with preeclampsia and hypertension seen when these conditions are present; Premature aging of villi, acute atherosis of maternal arteries, and obliterative changes in fetal stem arteries may occur

TABLE 8 Classification of Diabetes Mellitus in Pregnancy

Class	Criteria	Vascular disease
A_1	Gestational diabetes controlled by diet (fasting glucose <105 mg/dl)	None
A_2	Gestational diabetes requiring insulin for control (fasting glucose >105 mg/dl)	None
B	Onset after age 20 with <10 years' duration of diabetes	None
C	Onset before age 20 or 10–19 years' duration	None
D	Onset before age 10 or >20 years' duration	Retina
F	Onset at any age, of any duration, with nephropathy	Kidneys
R	Onset at any age, of any duration, with proliferative retinopathy	Retina
H	Onset at any age, of any duration, with arteriosclerotic heart disease	Heart disease
T	Onset at any age, of any duration, with renal transplant	

Placental lesions tend to be less severe and less frequent in gestational diabetes than in well-established diabetes.[117]

Abortion

Gross Features

Torsion, stricture, and true knots of the umbilical cord, massive subchorial thrombosis (Breus' mole), partial hydatidiform mole, and maternal floor infarction of the placenta have been described in abortion specimens.

Histologic Features

Fox[4] describes four histologic patterns of villous changes: (1) normal appearance; (2) fetal vascular obliteration, stromal fibrosis, and prominent syncytiotrophoblast and cytotrophoblast; (3) hydropic (or hydatidiform) villi with hypovascularity or avascularity; and (4) hypoplastic villi. Some authors use the terms "hydropic" and "hydatidiform change" synonymously, while others restrict the use of the term "hydatidiform change" to those cases in which there is trophoblastic hyperplasia. A spectrum of abnormalities extending from mere hydropic change to a full-fledged hydatidiform change with trophoblastic hyperplasia has also been described. I believe that the term "hydatidiform change" should be used only in the presence of trophoblastic hyperplasia. Hypoplastic villi are characterized by small size, deficient vascularity and a hypoplastic trophoblast.[4]

Hydropic villi without trophoblastic hyperplasia (in fact, the trophoblast is attenuated) is characteristic of hydropic abortus. This hydropic change involves virtually all villi. The biphasic pattern of normal villi admixed with hydropic villi seen in partial mole is absent in hydropic abortus.[118] In partial mole, the hydropic villi show circumferential trophoblastic proliferation.[119] Polar accentuation of the trophoblast seen in normal-first-trimester pregnancies is not sufficient for the diagnosis of partial mole.

Pathogenesis

The changes in pattern (2) above and the hydropic change in the villi are secondary to fetal death. When there is trophoblastic hyperplasia in association with the hydropic change in the villi, a diagnosis of partial hydatidiform mole is warranted. DNA analysis is essential to confirm the diagnosis of partial mole.[120] However, it should be noted that in a recent study, about 10% of cases of the hydropic abortus showed triplody, indicating that all triploid conceptions may not progress to partial mole.[121] Villous hypoplasia is found only in the placenta of abortuses showing heteroploidy.

Comment

A number of histologic classifications of villous changes in abortions described above have been proposed to explore the correlation with chromosomal abnormalities and with the outcome of future pregnancies. The reader is referred to the original articles for details.[119a,119b] Fox considers these classifications of little practical value.[119c]

Premature Labor and Delivery[122,123]

This complication can be associated with a number of obstetrical conditions (e.g., abruptio placentae, preeclampsia), maternal conditions (e.g., hypertension, chronic debilitating disease), or premature rupture of membranes occurring spontaneously or secondary to acute chorioamnionitis.[105,123] In many cases, there is no demonstrable associated, well-defined condition. The placental findings can be divided into two groups: (1) those related to the associated conditions listed above, which have been described in sections related to these conditions, and (2) those seen in prematurely delivered placentas in otherwise normal pregnancies. These findings are briefly described below.

Gross Features

The placenta is small in size and weight for the gestational age. The incidence of infarcts, perivillous fibrin deposition and calcification is less than in term placentas.

Histologic Features

The villi may have a maturity appropriate for the gestational age, may be fully mature,[122] or may show delayed maturation. There is a high incidence of fibrinoid necrosis of villi.

Pathogenesis

The abnormalities of villous maturity may be due to asynchrony between fetal and placental development. Excessive fibrinoid necrosis of villi may be related to immunologic phenomena of graft rejection. However, there is no firm evidence for this hypothesis.

Comment

The working group on indications for placental examination of the College of American Pathologists' Conference on the Examination of the Placenta has recommended examination of placentas from premature deliveries occurring before 32 weeks of gestation, although according to the conventional definition, an infant born at or before 37 weeks is considered premature. In many cases, no placental cause of premature labor and delivery can be found.

Postmaturity

"Postmaturity" is defined as a gestational age >42 weeks. It should be noted that some cases of postmaturity may be labeled as such due to incorrect calculation of the gestational period.

Gross Features

The placenta may be unusually heavy. Infarcts and calcification may be present, but these changes are not more severe or more frequent than those in term placentas. Other lesions such as perivillous fibrin deposition, retroplacental hematoma and fetal artery thrombosis also are not more frequent.

Histologic Features

The villi show stromal fibrosis, prominent syncytial knots, slight cytotrophoblastic proliferation, and trophoblastic basement membrane thickening. The fetal stem arteries may show obliterative endarteritis. Fox[4] describes four patterns of villous vascularity: (1) normovascular villi, (2) hypovascular but otherwise normal villi ("hypovascularity" is defined as constricted or collapsed capillaries), (3) normovascular villi with cytotrophoblastic hyperplasia and trophoblastic basement membrane thickening, and (4) hypovascular villi with the two abnormalities mentioned in (3) above. No pathologic lesion is seen in the maternal decidual arteries.

Pathogenesis

The changes have been considered as manifestations of placental senescence, a view that Fox disagrees with.[4] The lesions are probably related to hypoperfusion of the placental blood vessels because of fetal factors and to uteroplacental ischemia. However, the reasons for fetal hypoperfusion and uteroplacental ischemia occurring after term are not known. Factors such as fetal senescence, accumulation of vasoconstrictor mediators and reduction in maternal blood flow secondary to reduced fetal perfusion of villi have been implicated.[4]

Oligohydramnios and Polyhydramnios

Amniotic fluid provides the medium for free fetal movements and has a cushioning effect to prevent possible fetal injury. Secretion of amniotic epithelium and, from about the fourth month of gestation, fetal urine are the main sources of the amniotic fluid. Cellular and noncellular debris from the desquamated epithelial cells of the skin, respiratory tract, and urinary tract is also present. The amount of amniotic fluid at midpregnancy and at term is about 400 and 1000 ml, respectively. Marked reduction of amniotic fluid is defined as oligohydramnios. Amniotic fluid of >2000 ml is considered polyhydramnios.

Causes of oligohydramnios include (1) postmaturity, (2) urinary tract obstruction, (3) renal agenesis or severe bilateral renal cystic disease, and (4) chronic leakage due to prolonged rupture of membranes. Amnion nodosum, which has been described above, is the main lesion of the placenta in oligohydramnios. When there is chronic leakage of amniotic fluid due to prolonged rupture of membranes, ACA is present. Polyhydramnios is seen in association with (1) anomalies of the gastrointestinal tract (e.g., in esophageal atresia resulting in absence of swallowing of amniotic fluid) and of the central nervous system (e.g., in anencephaly resulting in transudation of fluid from exposed meninges), (2) monozygotic twin pregnancy with twin transfusion syndrome resulting in increased urine output of the recipient twin (the donor twin sac shows oligohydramnios), (3) maternal diabetes, and (4) chorangioma. The weight of the placenta tends to be high in polyhydramnios.

Premature, Preterm, and Prolonged Rupture of Membranes

The three terms used in relation to rupture of membranes have the following connotations: (1) "premature" indicates rupture before onset of labor at any gestational age, (2) "preterm" indicates rupture before 38 weeks' gestation, and (3) "prolonged" indicates rupture of more than 24 hours' duration. The rupture of membranes may be spontaneous, iatrogenic (attempt to induce labor) or secondary to ACA. ACA is being increasingly recognized as an important cause of premature and preterm rupture of membranes and preterm labor[105,123] (see the section on ACA above). In prolonged rupture of membranes occurring spontaneously, the amniotic cavity is exposed to the organisms in the genital tract. Therefore, the main placental lesion seen in all types of rupture of the membrane (premature, preterm and prolonged) is ACA. Abruptio placentae with or without demonstrable retroplacental hematoma tends to occur in patients with premature rupture of membranes.

Maternal Fever

When other causes of fever are ruled out, fever is the most reliable indicator of ACA. Therefore, one should look for this lesion in the placenta sent for pathologic examination. The organisms causing specific maternal infections that may or may not be identified definitively by the obstetrician can involve the placenta and its membranes and the fetus. The placental lesions in these infections include villitis, ACA, and funisitis. The organisms causing villitis, ACA and funisitis have been described in the respective sections above. Histopathologic examination of the placenta may provide the first definitive indication of a specific viral, bacterial, fungal, or parasitic infection so that appropriate measures can be taken for the management of the neonate. Malarial parasites may be present in maternal RBCs in the intervillous space in maternal malaria (Figure 55).

Maternal Substance Abuse

The substances of abuse include alcohol, cigarettes, cocaine, and heroin. Higher incidences of ACA, subnormal weight, villitis, abruptio placentae, and meconium staining have been described in alcohol abuse.[124] On the other hand, the placenta may be normal. Alcohol can move across the placenta to the fetus readily, resulting in IUGR and fetal alcohol syndrome. Reduced weight, hypovascularity, and stromal fibrosis of villi related to ischemic factors and a higher incidence of single umbilical artery have been described in placentas from mothers who smoke.[5] Ultrastructural and histomorphometric studies of the villi have demonstrated reduced trophoblastic elements.[125,126] A higher incidence of premature rupture of membranes and abruptio placentae has been described in mothers abusing cocaine.[127] ACA, meconium staining, and fetal growth retardation were the principal findings in the placentas of heroin-abusing mothers.[128] It should be noted that in the study of the correlation of placental lesions with substance abuse, there may be abuse of more than one substance by a mother and the social factors may determine the higher incidence of lesions such as ACA.

Abruptio Placentae

This clinical syndrome has been discussed above in the section on retroplacental hematoma.

Systemic Lupus Erythematous (SLE), Lupus Anticoagulant, and Anticardiolipin

Patients with SLE have lupus anticoagulant and anticardiolipin antibodies. It has been observed that these antibodies are present in patients with other clinical conditions or with no demonstrable disease. Anticardiolipin and lupus anticoagulant show cross-reactivity. Pregnant women having these antibodies, with or without SLE, show increased fetal loss. Abramowsky et al.[129] found one or more of the following lesions in the placenta from mothers with SLE: (1) infarcts (>25% of the placental volume), (2) acute atherosis of decidual maternal arteries, (3) retroplacental hemorrhages from rupture of damaged vessels, (4) premature aging of the villi, and (5) obliterative changes of the fetal stem arteries. Immunofluorescence studies showed deposits of C3, IgM, and fibrin in the decidual arteries. Acute atherosis with thrombosis of affected decidual arteries and placental infarction have also been described in mothers with lupus anticoagulant.[130] However, it should be noted that preeclampsia is common in SLE and more so in women with lupus nephritis. In such cases, it may be difficult to differentiate between preeclampsia and lupus nephritis and between eclampsia and SLE with neurologic manifestations (convulsions). Acute atherosis of decidual arteries alleged to occur in SLE may be related to supervening preeclampsia.

LESIONS OF THE PLACENTA IN FETAL DISORDERS (Table 9)

Multiple Births

Twin Births

Gross Features. Twin placentas may be partially or completely fused or may be entirely separate. The size of each placental territory should be measured. In some cases, the territories may be unequal. The partial fusion may

TABLE 9 Salient Features of Placenta in Fetal Disorders

Disorder	Salient gross features	Salient microscopic features	Comment
Twin birth with MoDi placenta	Single placental disc, two amniotic sacs, of same or dissimilar size, and dividing septum attached to the fetal surface are seen; velamentous or marginal insertion and a single umbilical artery are more frequent; vascular anastomoses are present in 85–100% of cases; pallor of the donor and congestion of the recipient territory are seen when there is twin transfusion syndrome; amnion nodosum may be present in the donor territory	Histologic findings reflecting the gross findings are seen; the dividing septum is composed of two amnions only, without intervening chorion	Superficial vascular anastomoses can be visualized by naked eye examination; injection studies may be done to confirm these findings; injection studies are the only way to demonstrate deeper arteriovenous anastomoses via a shared lobule (see text for details of methods); the twin transfusion syndrome is seen in 15–30% of twins with MoDi placenta
Twin birth with DiDi placenta	Two placental discs may be completely separate or fused, resembling the MoDi placenta; the fusion may be partial, with fusion of membranes, only or an intervening portion of the membranes between the two disks may be present; a dividing septum is present in fused placentas; vascular anastomoses are extremely rare	Dividing septum shows chorion between the two amnions	Twin transfusion is extremely rare; the pathology of separate DiDi placentas is same as that of singleton placenta

TABLE 9 (Continued)

Disorder	Salient gross features	Salient microscopic features	Comment
Twin birth with MoMo placenta	Only one amniotic sac and a single placental disk without a dividing septum are present; a small amniotic fold representing disrupted septum of a previously DiDi placenta may be present; vascular anastomoses are uncommon; findings of twin transfusion syndrome described above may be seen; the cords may be entangled	No specific features are seen	Demonstration of vascular anastomoses should be done when twin transfusion syndrome is present—this is the rarest type of twin placenta; a high incidence of fetal morbidity and mortality is present
Vanishing twins	Plaques of perivillous fibrin, embryonic remnants on the membranes, and a second amniotic sac, with or without an embryo, may be found; the embryonic remnant appears as a flattened yellow plaque, with or without occular pigment	The embryonic remnant shows autolyzed embryonic tissues	There are few reports describing the pathologic features of the placenta; the placenta should be carefully examined for detection of the embryonic remnant; the twin may be lost via vaginal bleeding
Fetus papyraceous/fetus compressus (FP/FC)	FP/FC representing a dead twin is identifiable as a plaque of dehydrated remnant, with or without identifiable fetal parts; umbilical cord torsion or massive infarction may cause fetal death	Histologic findings reflect the gross abnormalities; autolyzed fetal tissues are seen in the sections from FP/FC	Careful gross examination is essential to detect FP/FC—roentgenograms may be taken to show the skeleton of FP/FC; the cause of fetal death may not be evident

Acardiac twin	MoMo placenta with artery-to-artery and vein-to-vein anastomoses between the viable twin and acardiac twin placental territories	No specific microscopic features	Vascular anastomoses should be looked for; the acardiac twin has no heart or a severely malformed heart; other malformations may also be present
Intrauterine growth retardation (IUGR)	IUGR is associated with maternal factors (preeclampsia, chronic renal disease, substance abuse, etc.), fetal factors (severe congenital anomalies, chromosomal disorders, intrauterine infarction, etc.), and placental factors (extrachorial placenta, velamentous insertion of cord, maternal floor infarction, VUE, extensive infarction or perivillous fibrin deposition, etc.); placenta findings related to the maternal, fetal, and placental factors are seen	Histologic findings related to fetal, maternal, and placental factors are seen	The placenta is small, which is a reflection than a cause of IUGR; the cause of IUGR may not be evident, and the placenta may be normal except for its size
Erythroblastosis fetalis	Enlarged weight and size, pallor, intervillous thrombi	Villi: immature with persistent cytotrophoblast, numerous normoblasts in capillaries, villous edema, hemosiderin in chorionic macrophages	Severity of placental changes is related to severity of fetal anemia; the fetus is hydropic

TABLE 9 (Continued)

Disorder	Salient gross features	Salient microscopic features	Comment
Nonimmunologic hydrop fetalis (NIHF)	The causes of NIHF include genetic and metabolic disorders, chromosomal abnormalities, cardiac and pulmonary anomalies, thalassemia, fetomaternal hemorrhage, fetal infection, fetal tumors, arrhythmias, congenital nephrotic syndrome; placental findings related to the disorders are present	Histologic findings related to the associated condition are seen	In ~22% of NIHF cases, no associated condition can be found
Chromosomal disorders (trisomy 13, 18, 21)	Small placenta, high incidence of single umbilical artery	Villi: delayed maturation, hypovascularity, large, atypical Hofbauer or trophoblastic cells	Karyotyping should be done on the chorion or amnion
Metabolic disorders	Large hydropic placenta	Vacuoles in the syncytiotrophoblasts, intermediate trophoblast, Hofbauer cells, endothelium and fetal WBCs in the villous capillaries	The vacuoles represent the accumulated metabolite, which is dissolved during processing; electron microscopy may give clues regarding the precise diagnosis (e.g., Niemann–Pick disease, glycogenosis type IV); biochemical study of snap-frozen fresh placental tissue is essential for definitive demonstration of enzyme deficiency

Antepartum stillbirth, intrauterine fetal death (IUFD)	Massive infarction, retroplacental hematoma, large chorangioma, true knot, torsion or stricture of the cord, nuchal cord, intrauterine infection, maternal floor infarction, and extensive perivillous fibrin deposition are placental lesions that may lead to IUFD	Histologic findings reflecting these placental lesions are seen; assessment of the interval between IUFD and delivery can be made on the basis of histologic findings (see text for details)	Maternal conditions (e.g., preeclampsia) and fetal conditions (e.g., erythroblastosis fetalis) may also cause IUFD; certain placental abnormalities such as stromal fibrosis, hypovascularity, thrombosis of vessels in stem villi, and villous edema are secondary to IUFD; confined placental mosaicism may occur in rare cases (see text for details)

involve the membranes alone or may occur in combination with the placental disks. In completely fused placentas, there is a single disk with one or two amniotic sacs. When there are two amniotic sacs, the fetal surface of the fused placenta contains a septum composed of two amnions and chorions or two amnions alone, depending on whether the placenta is dichorionic diamniotic (DiDi) or monochorionic diamniotic (MoDi), respectively. The septum in the monochorionic placenta is thin and translucent, whereas that in the dichorionic fused placenta is thick and opaque. These features of the monozygotic twin placenta are determined by the timing of the duplication of the fertilized ovum and the site of the implantation of the two ova. Chorion and amnion are differentiated between 3 and 8 days and between 8 and 13 days after fertilization, respectively. Therefore, if duplication occurs at or before 3 days, the twin placenta wil be DiDi since each ovum will develop its own chorion and amnion. If the duplication occurs between 3 and 8 days, a MoDi placenta is the result since the ovum already has its chorion at the time of duplication, but the amnion will develop in each ovum separately after duplication. When duplication occurs between 8 and 13 days, the rare monochorionic monoamniotic (MoMo) placenta is seen since the ovum already has both the chorion and amnion before duplication. Conjoined twins are seen when duplication occurs at or after 13 days. The presence or absence and extent of fusion of monozygotic dichorionic or dizygotic twin placentas are determined by the sites of implantation of the duplicated fertilized ova or of the two separate ova. If the implantation sites are close to each other, there is fusion, the extent of which is determined by the closeness of the sites. If the implantation of the two ova occurs at sites which are far apart, two separate placentas will be present.

An important gross feature seen in 85–100% of MoDi placentas is the presence of vascular anastomoses between the two territories on either side of the septum (Figure 77). Such vascular anastomoses are extremely rare in dichorionic fused placentas and uncommon in MoMo placentas. There are two basic types of anastomosis: superficial and deep. The superficial anastomoses can be between two arteries or two veins or between an artery and a vein. The deep anastomoses are between an artery of one territory and a vein of the other territory indirectly through a shared placental lobule (Figure 78). In such an anastomosis, a lobule of one placental territory receives its arterial supply from its own territory, but the capillaries drain into the vein of the other territory. These shared lobules, which are variable in number, are usually present near the vascular equator of the fused placenta. The different shared lobules may have anastomoses in the same direction or in two different directions (i.e., an artery of twin A to a vein of twin B in some shared lobules and an artery of twin B to a vein of twin A in the remaining shared lobules) (Figure 78).

Demonstration of Vascular Anastomoses[5]

This can be done by macroscopic examination and injection studies. Most MoDi placentas have both superficial and deep anastomoses, and there may be more than one anastomosis of either type. In most instances, the superficial anastomoses are readily detected by the following procedure.[5] First, the fetal

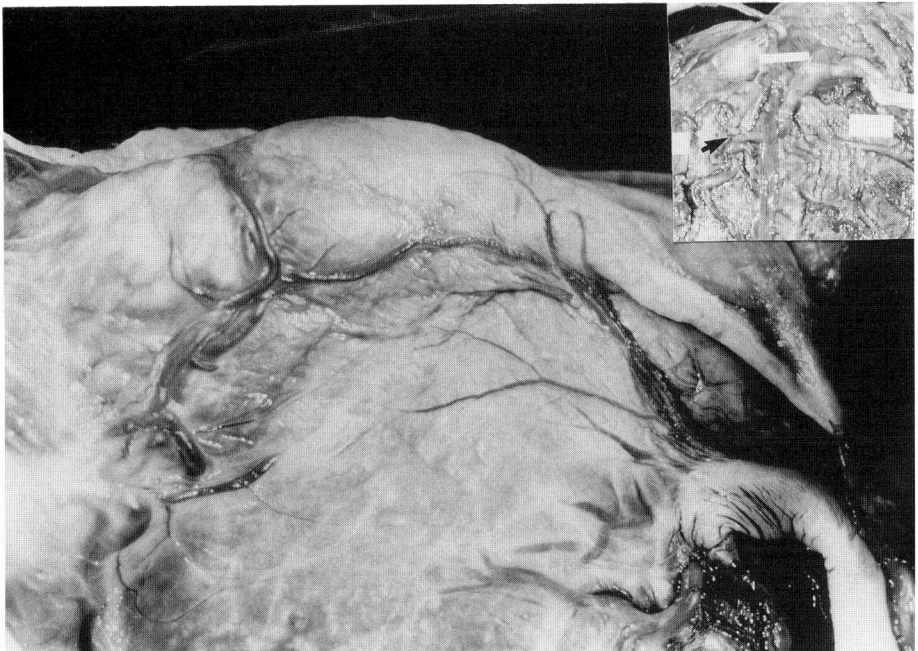

FIGURE 77. Fused MoDi placenta showing superficial artery-to-artery anastomosis between the two territories. The amnion and a portion of the septum have been stripped off for clearer demonstration of the anastomosis. The inset shows another similar specimen in which the septum and the amnion have not been stripped off. Note the artery of one territory (arrow) going underneath the septum and joining an artery in the opposite territory (arrow).

surface should be wiped clean and dry. Stripping of the amnion from the fetal surface (except at and near the dividing septum) results in better visualization of the blood vessels. The arteries are smaller than and superficial to the veins. Each major artery arising at the insertion site of one of the territories and coursing toward the equator (usually the dividing septum) should be carefully followed along its course, which usually ends at the equator, where it enters the deeper part of the chorionic disk. The corresponding vein emerges close to where the artery enters. The vein then courses toward the insertion site along the fetal surface. If there is anastomosis, an artery will be seen to cross to the opposite placental territory and anastomose directly with an artery of that territory. In the vein-to-vein anastomoses, a vein, instead of coursing toward the cord insertion site, crosses to the other placental territory and anastomoses with a vein. The clue to the probable presence of an indirect artery-to-vein anastomoses via the capillary network of a shared lobule is the absence of a vein accompanying an artery on the fetal surface. Similarly, a vein emerging from the fetal surface without an accompanying artery should also raise the suspicion of an anastomo-

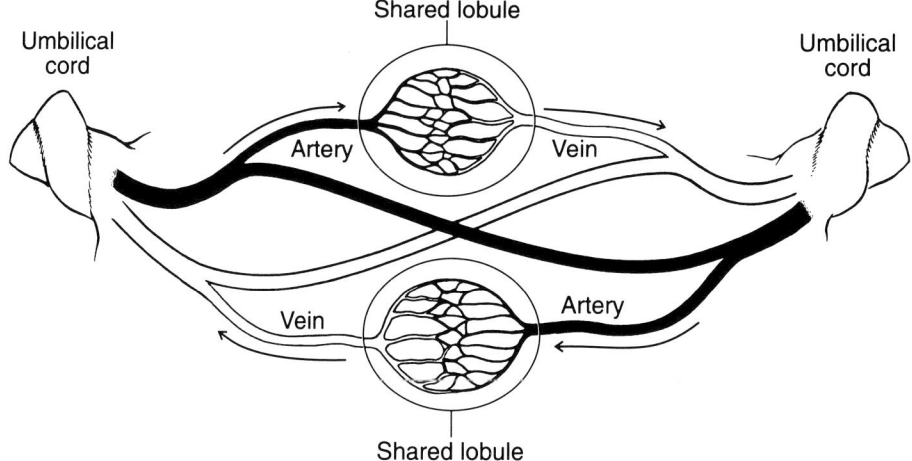

FIGURE 78. Diagrammatic representation of the vascular anastomoses in a twin placenta. Note that the deeper anastomoses via shared lobules may be in opposite directions. (Adapted from Benirschke K, Kaufmann P: *Pathology of the human placenta*, 2nd ed, Springer-Verlag, New York, 1990, Chap 25.)

sis via a shared lobule. Such an anastomosis cannot be seen by routine gross examination and requires injection studies for its demonstration.

The visual impression of superficial anastomoses and the suspicion of deep anastomoses may be confirmed by injection studies. Air, colored saline, milk, or dye can be used for these studies, which are done in the routine surgical pathology laboratory. Studies by injection of radiopaque dye or corrosion casts by injection of colored plastics require experience and special equipment and materials for their preparation and interpretation.[4,5,131] A routine injection study is performed by (1) inserting a needle in the blood vessel seen to be anastomosing with a vessel of the opposite territory, (2) injecting air or colored liquid, and (3) demonstrating the flow of the injected material into the other vessel. A photograph should be taken to document this injection study. The nature of the anastomosing vessels can be ascertained by the criteria mentioned above or by histologic study of the vessels. When colored saline or dye is injected through an artery or a vein (each of which is unaccompanied by a corresponding blood vessel), an area of one placental territory near the equator distends and becomes thicker in the placenta with deeper anastomoses. Eventually the colored saline or dye is seen to flow into a vessel of the opposite territory.[5] If as a result of the presence of anastomoses, there was twin transfusion syndrome (TTS) in a particular case (see below). The maternal and cut surfaces of the fused placental discs show a congested, turgid, blue-red appearance of the recipient territory, in marked contrast to the pale appearance of the donor territory (Figure 79). The other remarkable gross features of twin placentas include the higher incidence of single umbilical artery and velamentous insertion of the

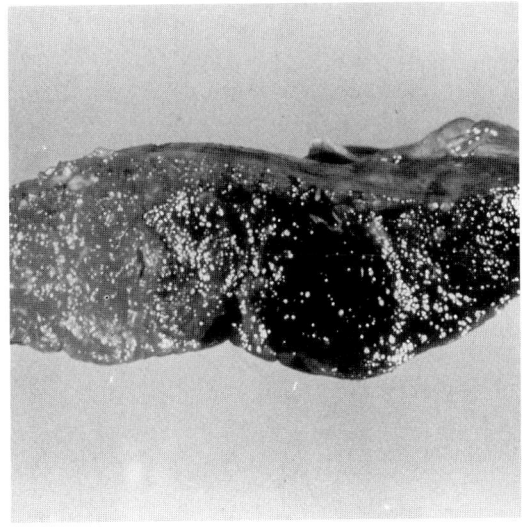

FIGURE 79. Cut surface of a MoDi placenta from a case of twin transfusion syndrome showing pallor of the donor territory and congestion of the recipient territory.

umbilical cord (Figure 80). The features of vanishing twin are described separately below.

Histologic Features

The sections made from the roll of the dividing septum and of the "T zone," i.e., the site of the chorionic plate to which the septum is attached perpendicularly, show the absence of chorion (Figure 81) or the presence of two fused chorions between the two amnions in monochorionic and dichorionic placentas, respectively. The sections taken from the blood vessels involved in the anastomoses reveal the true nature (i.e., arterial or venous) of the blood vessels. The histologic features of the various tissues from the two placental territories

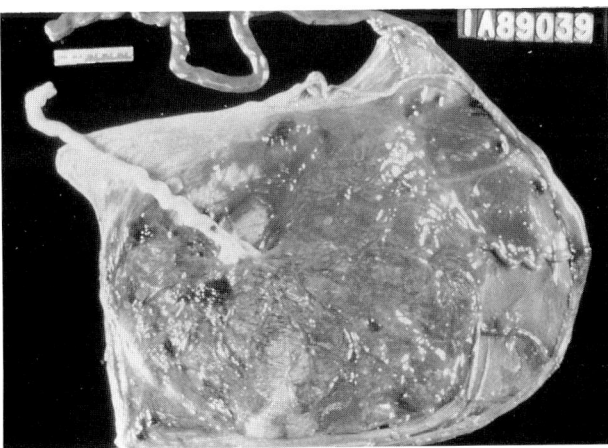

FIGURE 80. A MoMo twin placenta with velamentous insertion of one of the umbilical cords.

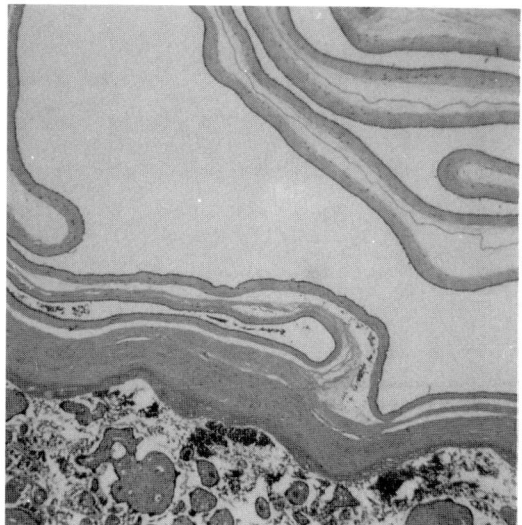

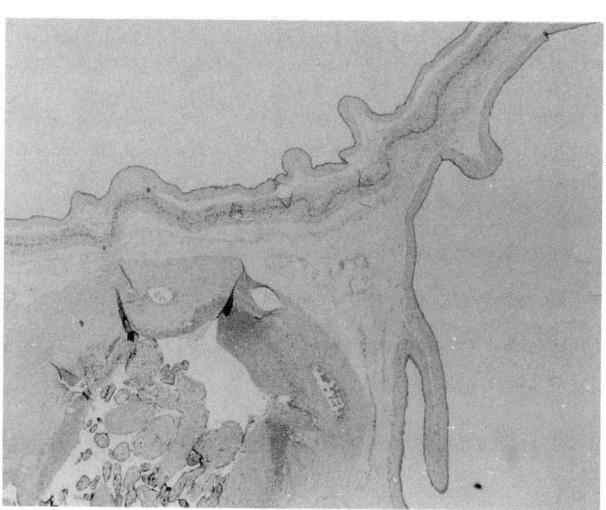

FIGURE 81. Dividing septum of (A) a MoDi placenta showing absence of chorion between the two amnions (H&E, ×40). (B) A dichorionic diamniotic (DiDi) placenta showing chorion between the two amnions (H&E, ×40).

show no difference in most cases. There are four exceptions: (1) In a dichorionic diamniotic (DiDi) placenta, only twin A may show ACA. (2) In a MoDi placenta with TTS, the villous capillaries of the recipient twin are markedly congested, whereas those of the donor twin are collapsed; in some cases there is marked edema or hydropic changes in the villi of the donor territory.[132] (3) Capillaries of the villi of the shared lobules (Figure 78) show presence of the injected dye when deeper arteriovenous anastomoses are present. (4) In the event of death of one of the twins, the placental villi of the territory of the dead twin show various abnormalities secondary to the fetal death (see the section on intrauterine fetal death below).

Significance of the Pathologic Examination of Twin Placentas. There are two main objectives of pathologic examination of twin placentas[4]: (1) to determine the type of placentation (mono- or dichorionic) and zygosity and (2) to demonstrate the vascular anastomoses. Monochorionic placentas are always monozygotic. Dichorionic placentas may be mono- or dizygotic. When there are two separate placental disks, the type of placentation is obviously dichorionic. Pathologic examination of these separate placentas is not helpful in determining the zygosity. The sex of the twins and other studies, such as blood group antigens if the sex of the twins is the same, are taken into consideration in determining the zygosity. Twins of the opposite sex are dizygotic and those of the same sex are either monozygotic or dizygotic. A monoamniotic placenta is monochorionic, and that of twins is monozygotic. When there is a fused (or single) placental disk with two amniotic sacs, it is necessary to determine whether the placenta is mono- or dichorionic. This is accomplished by histologic examination of the sections of the dividing septum and the T zone, as described above. If the fused placenta is monochorionic, the twins are monozygotic, but if it is dichorionic, the twins may be mono- or dizygotic. Demonstration of a deep arteriovenous anastomosis is helpful when TTS is suspected.

Since anastomoses are extremely rare in dichorionic placentas, it may be inferred that a placenta showing such anastomoses is most likely to be monochorionic. This indirect conclusion is necessary when the septum and T zone between the two territories are disrupted and a satisfactory histologic examination cannot be done to determine whether the placenta is mono- or dichorionic.

Comment. The methods of demonstration of vascular anastomoses have been described above. It should be emphasized that the deep arteriovenous anastomoses via the shared lobules are the most significant ones in TTS.[4,5,131] Although most MoDi twin placentas have both visually demonstrable superficial anastomoses between large blood vessels and deep anastomoses,[4,132] in some instances of TTS the former may be absent. Demonstration of deep anastomoses by the injection method, as described above, would be required in such cases.

It should be noted that the two territories of the fused twin placenta may not be delineated by the dividing septum if the septum is not inserted at the vascular equator. The vascular equator, which is represented by a perpendicular line drawn at the center of the line joining the sites of insertion of the two umbilical cords, delineates the two placental territories. The anastomosing blood vessels are seen to cross the vascular equator.

If the anastomoses are clearly visible on gross examination of the fetal surface, an injection study does not add significantly to their evaluation. Deeper anastomoses can be demonstrated only by injection studies, which require careful methodology and experience. Sections should be taken from the vascular equator of the fused twin placentas. In addition, sections from the two placental territories should be labeled separately. Histologic demonstration of the injected dye in the capillaries of the shared lobule and in the veins of the stem villi of the opposite placental territory is considered consistent with the presence of deeper arteriovenous anastomoses. Clearly visible or subtle but definite pallor of one territory, in contrast to the congestion of the other territory (Figure 79), is considered evidence of significant blood flow through deeper anastomoses. It is imperative that the obstetrician provide clinical details regarding the differences in birth weight and hematocrit of the twins when twin transfusion syndrome is suspected. The pathologist can demonstrate the presence of anastomoses, but whether clinically significant blood flow has occurred across the anastomoses is determined only by the differences in the birth weight and hematocrit of the twins and in the color of the two placental territories.

Types of Placentas in Twin Pregnancy

Monochorionic Diamniotic (MoDi) Placenta

Incidence. MoDi placentas are present in about 30% of twin pregnancies.

Gross Features. MoDi placenta has, by definition, a single placental disk and two amniotic sacs. The dividing septum between the two sacs is attached to the fetal surface. The site of attachment of the thin, translucent septum may be the same as or different from that of the vascular equator. The latter represents a line drawn at right angles at the midpoint of the line joining the insertion sites of the umbilical cords. The two amniotic sacs may be the same size or of different sizes. Single umbilical artery and marginal or velamentous insertion of the umbilical cord are more frequent in MoDi placentas than in singleton placentas. Most of the MoDi placentas have superficial and deep anastomoses. There may be oligohydramnios in the amniotic sac of the donor twin in cases of TTS. Amnion nodosum may be seen in that sac. In TTS there may be intrauterine death of one or both twins. The blood vessels on the fetal surface should be carefully examined for the presence of vascuar anastomoses and injection studies carried out as described above. Pallor of the donor territory and congestion of the recipient territory are seen on the maternal and cut surfaces in cases of TTS (Figure 79).

Histologic Features. The dividing septum is composed of two amnions only (Figure 81). In the cases of TTS, capillaries of the villi of the donor territory are collapsed, and those of the recipient twin are congested.

Clinical Significance. Although vascular anastomoses are present in most MoDi placentas, it should be emphasized that TTS occurs in only a minority (15–30%) of these placentas.[4] The basic feature of TTS is transfer of blood from one twin (donor) to the other twin (recipient) via the deep arteriovenous anastomoses in the shared lobules. The anastomoses may be in the same (twin A to twin B) direction or in different (A to B and B to A) directions. The anastomoses in the opposite direction may compensate for each other. The artery-to-artery and vein-to-vein anastomoses may be balanced since the blood pressure in the two anastomosing blood vessels may be the same. It is conceivable that differences in the blood pressures of the two twins may make balanced, i.e., nonfunctional, artery-to-artery or vein-to-vein anastomosis functional. When the anastomoses are in the same direction and these anastomoses are small, clinically insignificant amounts of blood may be transferred from the arterial side (donor twin) to the venous side (recipient twin) of the anastomoses. However, when the anastomoses are large, TTS may become manifest. As indicated above, the most significant anastomoses are the deep anastomoses through the shared lobule(s).[133] All of the vascular anastomoses are formed during the early angiogenic phase of development of the placenta. But if they

Table 10 Ultrasonographic Criteria for Twin Transfusion Syndrome

1. Striking discrepancy in sizes of twins
2. Polyhydramnios surrounding the larger twin
3. Oligohydramnios surrounding the smaller twin (stuck-twin sign)
4. Monochorionic placenta
5. Same sex of twins

(The presence of adult RBCs in the circulation of the recipient twin after transfusion of such cells into the donor twin by cordocentesis has been used as a definitive criterion by some investigators.)

Adapted from Bruner JP, Rosemond RL. *Am J Obstet Gynecol* 169:925–930, 1993.

become functional, it occurs insidiously later in pregnancy or, in rare instances, acutely during labor and delivery. The latter timing is related to changes in the blood pressure consequent on uterine contractions.[133–135]

Clinically, TTS is diagnosed when the difference in hemoglobin levels and in birth weights of the donor and recipient twin is >5 g and 20%, respectively (see tables 10 and 11).[133] The donor generally has the lower values of hemoglobin and birth weight (Figure 82). Oligohydramnios in the donor twin with a "stuck" appearance on ultrasound and polyhydramnios in the recipient twin should suggest the possibility of TTS. In the acute variant of TTS, only the hemoglobin levels are markedly different. It should be emphasized that not all cases in which there are differences between hemoglobin levels and birth weights of the twins necessarily represent classical examples of TTS. The difference in birth weights may be due to velamentous insertion of the cord in one of the twins. The difference in the hemoglobin levels may be due to different techniques of cord clamping or death unrelated to TTS of one twin earlier than the other so that blood flows from the living twin to the dead twin.[136] Cerebral necrosis may occur in the donor twin as a result of TTS.[137] It has been suggested that in the event of death of one of the twins, thromboplastic material from the tissues of the dead fetus may pass into the circulation of the living fetus through the anastomoses, resulting in disseminated intravascular coagulation.[138] However, it is unlikely that the blood from the dead twin could be transfused into the living twin in the absence of any circulation in the former and against the gradient of higher intravascular pressure in the latter.[136]

Zygosity Twins of a MoDi placenta are always monozygotic.

Table 11 Neonatal Criteria for Diagnosis of Twin Transfusion Syndrome

1. Demonstration of vascular anastomoses between two placental territories
2. Intertwin hemoglobin difference of >5 g/dl*
3. Intertwin birth weight difference of >20%†

*Compensatory reticulocytosis in the donor twin may reduce the discrepancy between the hemoglobin concentrations.
†Acute intrapartum twin transfusions are not associated with a discrepancy in birth weights.
Adapted from Bruner JP, Rosemond RL. *Am J Obstet Gynecol* 169:925–930, 1993.

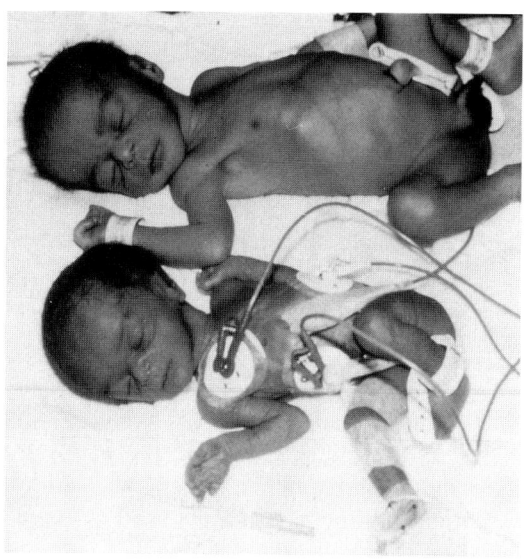

FIGURE 82. Twin transfusion syndrome, with the donor twin being pale and small and the recipient twin being plethoric and large. (Courtesy of Dr. Shyan Sun)

Dichorionic Diamniotic (DiDi) Placenta

Gross Features. The two placental disks may be entirely separate or intimately fused, resembling MoDi placenta. The pathology of separate DiDi placentas is the same as that of singleton placentas. The fusion may be partial, so that only the membranes fuse at or near the central portion of the placenta, the disks being separate. Alternatively, the disks may be connected by intervening membranes. The dividing membranous septum between the intimately fused DiDi placentas is thick and opaque. Vascular anastomoses are extremely rare.[139]

Histologic Features. The dividing membranous septum of the intimately fused DiDi placenta shows chorion between the two amnions. In some instances, the chorion extends from the chorionic plate of one of the two placental territories (as shown in Figure 81B), while in others, the chorions from the two placental territories extend into the dividing septum. The pathogenesis and significance of these two different structural aspects of the dividing septum of DiDi placenta are not known.

Clinical Significance. TTS is extremely rare in fused DiDi placentas.[139]

Zygosity. The twins of DiDi placentas can be mono or dizygotic.

Monochorionic Monoamniotic (MoMo) Placenta

Gross Features. This is the least common type of twin placenta. There is only one amniotic sac. Consequently there is no dividing septum on the fetal surface (Figure 80). However, in occasional cases, a small amniotic fold may be present along the fetal surface. It may represent a breakdown of a previously intact complete septum of what was a diamniotic placenta. There is a single placental disk. Vascular anastomoses are much less common than in MoDi placentas. The reason for the lesser frequency is not clear. However, it is possible that some of the MoMo placentas may represent completely fused DiDi placentas with total disruption and subsequent disappearance of the dividing septum.

Histologic Features. The fold that may be present on the fetal surface is composed of amnion. If one of the twins dies, in utero, the corresponding placental tissue becomes atrophic, or its circulation may persist via the anastomoses with the blood vessels of the surviving twin.

Clinical Significance. Because of fetal movements, the two umbilical cords can become entangled, leading to a high incidence of intrauterine death or perinatal morbidity of one or both twins. TTS is responsible for only a small minority of fetal deaths.

Vanishing Twins (VT)

This term is used to indicate the birth of a single child to a mother in whom sonographic diagnosis of multiple pregnancy was made during the first 15 weeks of gestation.[140] This phenomenon occurs in both natural pregnancies and pregnancies following in vitro fertilization. There are few reports of pathologic examination of the placenta.[141] Plaques of perivillous fibrin deposition, with or without embryonic remnants on the membranes, have been described by Jauniaux et al.[141] Evidence of a second sac, with or without a small embryo, may be found.[5] The embryo may appear as a flattened tan, yellow plaque, with or without ocular melanin. Vaginal bleeding occurs frequently in early pregnancy in patients with VT. It is possible that the VT may be aborted during one of these events. Pathologic examination of the placenta will fail to reveal the twin in such cases. It is imperative that the placenta and the membranes be carefully examined for the presence of a second sac and the remnants of a dead embryo in the cases of VT. The cause of the demise of the embryo/fetus is seldom clear. It is possible that it has an abnormal karyotype.

Fetus Papyraceus/Fetus Compressus (FP/FC)

FP/FC and VT form a continuum. In FP/FC one of the twin dies and is identifiable as a plaque composed of the compressed, dehydrated remnant of the dead fetus or of some identifiable fetal parts. This plaque may be missed if a careful gross examination is not done. A roentgenogram of the plaque will demonstrate the skeleton of the fetus (Figure 83). The placenta may be mono- or dichorionic. The death of the FP/FC may be due to umbilical cord torsion or massive infarction of its placenta.[5] The cause of fetal death may not be demonstrable in every case. Congenital anomalies may be present in FP/FC. Retention of FC/FC for a long time may lead to calcification (lithopedion).

Acardiac Twin

A specimen of acardiac twin may be submitted with the placenta. This represents a severely malformed monozygotic twin (or one of higher multiple birth). The heart is absent or only remnants of it are present. The critical factor in the continued growth and intrauterine viability of the acardiac twin is the presence of artery-to-artery and vein-to-vein anastomoses in a MoMo placenta. These anastomoses act as conduits for perfusion and return of blood from and to the cotwin with a normally formed heart. Without such anastomoses the twin

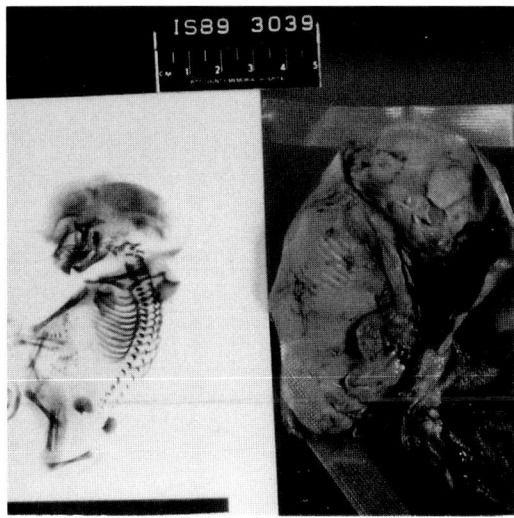

FIGURE 83. FP. Note the flattened dead fetus. Whole-body x-ray shows the skeleton of the fetus.

would vanish. The acardiac twin may show malformations of various organs ranging from their absence to complex anomalies. Liver has not been demonstrated in the acardiac twin.[5] The acardiac twin may be hydropic. Polyhydramnios of its sac may also occur. An x-ray of the acardiac twin should be obtained. Cord entanglement may occur since the placenta is MoMo.

Conjoined Twins (Siamese Twins)

These are rare (1 in 50,000 births). The placenta is usually MoMo. There may be separate or fused umbilical cords. The number of umbilical arteries and veins may be abnormal. The extent and body region of fusion of the two twins are variable (cephalopagus, thoracopagus, rachipagus, cephalothoracopagus, xiphopagus, ischiopagus, pygopagus). For the details of terminology and subtypes, the reader is referred to the review article by Harper et al.[142] and to the textbook by Potter and Craig.[143] The majority of conjoined twins are female. There is a high rate of stillbirth (or abortion) in conjoined twins, which may be submitted as a surgical pathology specimen along with the placenta. Depending on the type of conjoined twin, the different regions and organs of the body may be entirely separate or variably fused. Congenital anomalies may also be present within the separate or fused organs. Conjoined twins may also be found in triplet pregnancy.

Triplet and Multiple Births

Triplet pregnancy may be monzygotic (a single ovum replicating into two zygotes, with subsequent replication of one of these two zygotes), dizygotic, or trizygotic. The placenta may show various combinations, such as MoMo, MoDi, MoTri, and DiMo to TriTri. The placentas are frequently fused, but one or all three placentas may be separate. Similar combinations of structure are shown by the placenta of higher multiple births. The placental and fetal abnormalities described in relation to twin pregnancy can also occur in triplet and higher multiple births.

Intrauterine Growth Retardation (IUGR)

IUGR (small for dates/gestational age, inappropriate for dates/gestational age) is defined as a birth weight below the 10th percentile for the gestational age. It is different from prematurity (<37 weeks' gestation), low birth weight (LBW) (<2500 g), very LBW (<1500 g), or extremely LBW (<1000 g). IUGR may be related to the following:

1. *Maternal factors:* For example, preeclampsia, severe malnutrition, chronic renal disease with hypertension, maternal substance abuse.
2. *Fetal factors:* Severe congenital anomalies, chromosomal disorders, intrauterine infection (e.g., CMV, toxoplasmosis).
3. *Placental factors:* Lesions such as extrachorial placenta, marginal and velamentous insertion of the umbilical cord, maternal floor infarct, multiple infarcts (usually involving more than 30% of the placenta), extensive perivillous fibrin deposition, VUE, severe subchorionic fibrin deposition (>1 cm thickness involving >50% of the undersurface of the chorionic plate), large chorangioma, etc.[6] In rare instances of IUGR, acute atherosis of the decidual maternal arteries in the absence of sustained hypertension has been described.[112] The cause of IUGR cannot be determined in many cases. The small size of the placenta in IUGR is a reflection of generalized growth disturbance of the fetus, since the placenta is a fetal organ. Placental lesions related to the maternal and fetal factors described above are present.

Histologic examination of the placenta shows one of the following features in the villi:[4,6] (1) villous hypovascularity with stromal fibrosis and prominence of syncytial knots indicative of poor fetal perfusion, (2) cytotrophoblastic hyperplasia and thickening of trophoblastic basement membrane indicative of placental ischemia, (3) embryonic villi and villi with arrested branching indicative of delayed maturation, and (4) normal villi. When there is preeclampsia or hypertension, maternal arteries in the decidua show acute atherosis and arteriosclerosis, respectively.

Erythroblastosis Fetalis (EF)

EF is caused by Rh isoimmunization (Rh-negative mother with an Rh-positive fetus) and, rarely, by sensitization against other antigens (e.g., Kell) and ABO incompatibility. With the wide use of RhoGam, the incidence of EF has been markedly reduced. However, rare cases of Rh isoimmunization in missed, threatened, or full-fledged abortions in which there is lack of medical care still occur. In EF there is often hydrops fetalis. The placenta shows enlarged weight and size and pallor. The villi appear immature, with a persistent cytotrophoblast and prominent Hofbauer cells. There are numerous normoblasts in the villous capillaries. The villous stroma is edematous. Intervillous thrombi are present in about 30% of the placentas. Hemosiderin is seen occasionally in the chorionic macrophages. Hypoalbuminemia or fetal cardiac failure resulting from severe anemia is the cause of hydrops fetalis and of the placental changes in EF. The severity of placental changes is related to the severity of fetal anemia.

Placenta in Nonimmunologic Hydrops Fetalis

EF produces "immunologic" hydrops associated with an antigen–antibody reaction due to Rh isoimmunization or other factors. However, hydrops fetalis may also be seen in association with a nonimmunologic disease process. These include genetic metabolic disorders, chromosomal abnormalities, cardiac and pulmonary malformations, thalassemia, chronic fetomaternal hemorrhage, fetal infection (particularly human parvovirus B19 infection), fetal tumors (neuroblastoma, teratoma, leukemia, etc.), arrhythmias, congenital neophrotic syndrome, etc.[144] In ~22% of the cases of hydrops fetalis the cause is not known (idiopathic hydrops fetalis). Hydropic changes of variable severity are seen in the placenta in these conditions. In congenital neuroblastomas and leukemia, the tumor cells, along with normoblasts, are seen in the villous capillaries. In other conditions no specific diagnostic placental findings are present, and it is impossible to distinguish between immune and nonimmune hydrops on the basis of placental examination.

Chromosomal Disorders

In trisomies 13, 18, and 21 the placenta tends to be too small for the gestational age (the fetus also shows IUGR). A high incidence of SUA is noted in trisomies. Histologically, the villi show delayed maturation, with decreased vascularity and the presence of large, atypical cells in the stroma. The origin of these cells is not clear. They may represent Hofbauer cells or migrating trophoblast. In monosomy 45,X the villi show variable cellularity and stromal fibrosis. There is trophoblastic hypoplasia with deficient syncytial budding. The placental changes seen in triploidy have been described above. In tetraploidy similar changes are seen.

Metabolic Disorders

Placental changes have been described in gangliosidoses, mucopolysacharidoses, mucolipidoses, Gaucher's disease, Nieman–Pick disease, Wolman's disease, Zellweger syndrome, glycogen storage disease type II, ceroid lipofuscinosis, etc. On gross examination the placenta (and the fetus) may be hydropic. The accumulated metabolites in these disorders are soluble in water or xylene. Therefore, in routinely processed sections of the placenta, empty vacuoles are seen in syncytiotrophoblast, intermediate trophoblast, Hofbauer cells, endothelium, and fetal WBCs in the villous capillaries. Specific diagnosis of the metabolic disorder is not possible on the basis of histologic examination of the placenta alone.[145] Ultrastructural examination can be helpful. Jones et al. have described ultrastructural features of placentas and chorionic villus biopsies from a variety of metabolic disorders.[146] For example, characteristic ultrastructural features such as myelin bodies in Niemann–Pick disease and intralysosomal glycogen accumulation is glycogen storage disease, type II, were seen in a variety of placental cells. The authors emphasize the need for prompt fixation of the specimen for electron microscopy to avoid artifacts. Since biochemical investigation of the fresh tissue is essential for demonstration of the enzyme defect, a portion of fresh placental tissue should be snap frozen for these studies. Prenatal diagnosis of type II glycogenosis can be made by ultrastructural examination of amniotic cells obtained by amniocentesis.[147]

Antepartum Intrauterine Death with Retention and Maceration of the Fetus

Pathologic examination of the placenta is an integral part of the autopsy examination of the stillborn fetus. There are three types of placental findings: (1) placental lesions that cause intrauterine fetal death, (2) lesions related to maternal and fetal diseases that are the cause of fetal demise, and (3) placental lesions that are secondary to fetal death. In the first category are lesions such as massive infarction, retroplacental hematoma, large chorangioma, true knot, torsion and stricture of umbilical cord, nuchal cord, and intrauterine infection. These are not common but, when present, provide the explanation for fetal death. In rare cases, the stillbirth (or IUGR) may be associated with confined placental mosaicism (CPM).[148,149] CPM is characterized by a discrepancy between the fetal and placental karyotypes. Such a discrepancy is observed in 1–2% of pregnancies. The chromosomal abnormality may be confined to the cytotrophoblast or the placental stroma or both. The karyotype of the fetus may be normal or abnormal. The abnormality of the placental karyotype involves trisomy 2, 3, 8, 9, or 16. The significance of CPM in fetal development is not known. It has been suggested that it may interfere with placental function and may affect fetal growth and survival. Karyotyping should be done on cultured cells obtained from chorionic villous sampling and not from amniotic fluid. (In amniotic cells there is an admixture of fetal cells.) The placenta in CPM may not show any specific morphologic abnormalities on routine examination. In the second category are lesions related to maternal diseases such as preeclampsia and maternal hypertension (retroplacental hematoma and acute atherosis and/or arteriosclerosis of decidual uteroplacental maternal arteries) and fetal diseases such as EF and congenital anomalies with IUGR.

After fetal death, the placenta remains viable since the villi receive their oxygen and nutrients from the maternal circulation in the intervillous space. However, there is cessation of fetal circulation, which results in the following lesions: (1) progressive sclerosis of blood vessels in the stem villi followed by obliteration, (2) thrombosis of veins in the stem villi, (3) hypovascularity followed by stromal fibrosis of terminal villi, (4) an increased number of syncytial knots, and (5) villous edema. In addition, cytotrophoblastic hyperplasia and trophoblastic basement membrane thickening secondary to uteroplacental ischemia are seen since there is a reduction in maternal blood flow after fetal death. It is possible that villous "pulse", which is a factor in the circulation of blood through the intervillous space, is lost due to fetal demise. Thus there may be stagnation of maternal blood and a rise in pressure in the intervillous space. The net result is reduced maternal blood flow.[4] Focal calcification of villi, particularly of the trophoblastic basement membrane, is frequently seen. The main importance of knowledge of these placental changes is that these should not be considered as the cause of IUFD.

The placental changes described above commence within a few to several hours and are well established 5–6 days after IUFD. Genest[150] recently attempted to assess the interval between IUFD and birth on the basis of histologic changes in the placenta. He has shown that (1) villous intravascular karyorrhexis (of fetal normoblasts) is seen at ≥6 hours after IUFD, (2) fibroblastic septation of the lumen resembling recanalization of a thrombus and total luminal obliteration (due to fibromuscular hyperplasia) of blood vessels of stem villi are seen focally at ≥2 days and extensively at ≥2 weeks after IUFD, and (3) extensive fibrosis of terminal villi occurs at ≥2 or more weeks after IUFD. These correlations need to be confirmed by other retrospective and prospective studies.

Intrapartum Fetal Death

In contrast to antepartum fetal death, there is no maceration in the fetus and there is insufficient time for any of the postfetal death placental changes to occur. The placenta may be normal or may show lesions such as retroplacental hematoma, velamentous insertion of the umbilical cord with or without rupture of the vasa previa (the membranous vessels coursing over the internal os), nuchal cord, and true knot of the cord. Placenta previa and placenta accreta may also be associated with intrapartum stillbirth.

IATROGENIC LESIONS OF THE PLACENTA, UMBILICAL CORD, AND MEMBRANES

A number of diagnostic and therapeutic procedures including amniocentesis, umbilical cord blood sampling and intraperitoneal and intravascular fetal transfusion may be done during pregnancy. Ultrasound guidance is used for localization of the placenta and umbilical cord. In rare instances, traumatic lesions such as small lacerations of the fetal surface of the placenta of the blood vessels on the fetal surface and the umbilical cord itself may occur. Hemorrhage occurs at the site(s) of laceration with or without hematoma formation (Figure 84). The hemorrhage may extend underneath the amnion or into the amniotic cavity if a surface blood vessel is ruptured.

Intraamniotic bleeding, with or without an umbilical cord hematoma, is seen when the umbilical cord vessel is ruptured.[151] The fetal surface of the placenta, the blood vessels of the umbilical cord, and their branches along the

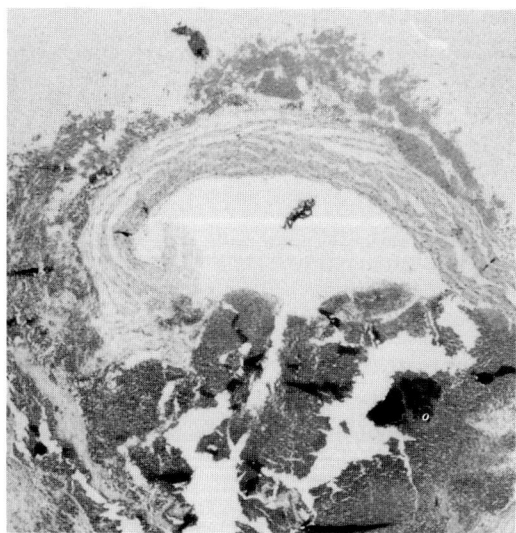

FIGURE 84. Disruption of the umbilical vein with formation of a hematoma secondary to fetal intravascular transfusion (H&E, ×40).

fetal surface should be carefully examined to detect the laceration(s). It should be noted that lacerations of the fetal surface of the placenta may also result in transplacental fetal bleeding into the mother. Premature delivery and intrauterine death may occur following these procedures. The clinician should provide an adequate history of any obstetric diagnostic and therapeutic procedures performed during pregnancy so that the pathologist can look specifically for iatrogenic lesions.

TRAUMATIC LESIONS OF THE PLACENTA

Abdominal trauma (of which automobile accident is one of the most common causes) can result in placental abruption and transplacental fetal bleeding. Retroplacental hematoma may be present. Contusion and tears of the placenta may lead to bleeding into the amniotic sac.[5,152] Bruises of the villous tissue with severe intravillous hemorrhage can also occur.[5] Concurrent fetal injuries including skull fractures, with or without cranial hemorrhages, have also been described.

PLACENTA IN PREGNANCIES AFTER IN VITRO FERTILIZATION (IVF) AND EMBRYO TRANSFER (ET)

Gavriil et al.[153] compared placental morphologic features of 70 singleton, 20 twin, and 10 multiple pregnancies occurring after IVF and ET with 70 placentas from spontaneous singleton pregnancies and 20 placentas from spontaneous twin pregnancies. The frequency of bilobate and succenturiate placentas was significantly higher in the IVF/ET singleton pregnancies ($p < 0.025$). The mean distance between the site of cord insertion and the closest placental margin was significantly shorter in the IVF/ET group (3.19 vs. 4.62 cm) ($p < 0.001$). In twin pregnancies no significant differences between the placental morphologic features of the two groups were observed. However, multiple pregnancies occurring after IVF/ET were complicated by the vanishing twin phenomenon. In some cases, multiple pregnancies were artificially reduced.

The abnormalities of placental shape in the singleton pregnancy after IVF/ET may be related to (1) interference with proper orientation of the blastocyst when it is attached to the endometrium or (2) superficial implantation. The near-marginal insertion of the umbilical cord may be associated with oblique orientation of the blastocyst in pregnancy occurring after IVF/ET or with abnormalities of the uterus such as leiomyomas, endometriosis, or sequelae of pelvic inflammatory disease seen not infrequently in mothers requiring IVF/ET to become pregnant. Remnant embryos which could not be demonstrated in any of the cases of vanishing twin phenomenon were present in the cases of multiple pregnancy with artificial reduction.

SPECIMENS RELATED TO PLACENTAL LASER SURGERY

Placental laser surgery which is not an established and widely used procedure, can be attempted to treat placental pathologic lesion(s) which produce fetal morbidity, or threaten to produce fetal mortality. Twin transfusion in monochorionic twins, acardiac twinning and chorangioma are the three placental lesions which can be potentially treated by occluding the placental blood vessels which connect the circulations of the twins in the former two conditions or those supplying the chorangioma (154). The neodymium-YAG laser produces coagulation rather than vaporization of the tissues at 60 to 90°. Immediate occlusion of blood vessels and finally scar formation are seen in the affected tissues. De Lia and his colleagues have described the results of three cases of twin transfusion syndrome treated by laser surgery (155). The anastomosing blood vessels at the vascular equator on the fetal surface are treated by the laser. Whitish-tan scars containing occluded anastomosing blood vessels are seen at the vascular equator on the fetal surface when the pathologist subsequently examines the placenta after delivery. Sections for histologic examination should be taken from the scars.

COMMENT

As indicated in the Introduction, the placenta is not a favorite subject of surgical pathologists. Unlike other areas of surgical pathology, precise pathologic diagnosis of a placental abnormality seldom has a direct and immediate clinical impact. Pathologic examination of the placenta is often regarded by the obstetrician as one more way of documenting or confirming a maternal or fetal disorder that has been suspected or diagnosed on the basis of clinical features, laboratory data, and imaging techniques. However, there are definite instances in which pathologic examination of the placenta has immediate or remote but direct clinical implications. For example, an infection (listeriosis, group B streptococcal chorioamnionitis, villitis due to CMV, or *Toxoplasma gondii*) may first be detected on placental examination. Appropriate therapy may then be instituted immediately, or, if there has been a stillbirth, appropriate steps to prevent poor outcome may be taken in a subsequent pregnancy. In occasional cases, a definite cause of intrauterine fetal death can also be ascertained from the placental examination. Medicolegal importance of placental pathology in specific situations, such as perinatal asphyxia and death of one of the twins, has been emphasized in the literature.

However, in many placentas sent to the surgical pathologist because of the presence of maternal or fetal disorders, the placenta may be normal or may show findings of the same degree of severity as seen in some normal placentas. Thus the placental examination is inconclusive and noncontributory. The occurrence of many of the gross and microscopic lesions in normal placentas is often frustrating to the surgical pathologist, who may not have the time or the tools to carry out the quantitative histomorphometric studies that are reported in the literature. Further, in many instances, even the histomorphometric studies may be inconclusive (e.g., in maternal diabetes). Moreover, the knowledge that fetal artery thrombosis is seen in 4.5% of normal placentas and 10% of diabetic placentas does not help in the interpretation of the significance of that finding in an individual placenta without the benefit of a clinical history. I recommend to the surgical pathologist the following approach in dealing with placentas:

1. Develop a list of indications for the pathologic examination of the placenta in consultation with the obstetrician and neonatologist.
2. Only those placentas satisfying the guidelines in the list of indications should be sent to the surgical pathology laboratory. If there is a full-time perinatal pathologist on staff or if there is a specific research interest, placentas from all deliveries may be sent.
3. Familiarize yourself with the normal gross and microscopic anatomy of the placenta by studying a few normal placentas, diagrams, and a set of histology slides that represent all the obvious and less obvious histologic components of a normal placenta (e.g., yolk sac remnant, cytotrophoblast, cell islands of intermediate trophoblast). (Figures 1–20) (section on the structure of the placenta).
4. The normal range of the gross and microscopic lesions of the placenta should be kept in mind while interpreting the findings and making a diagnosis. For example, placental infarcts occupying <5% of the placental volume should be recorded in the gross and microscopic description, but a pathologic diagnosis of a placental infarct of this extent may not be given in the report since placental infarct(s) involving <5% of the placental surface can be seen in normal placentas.
5. Quantitative assessment of the extent of involvement of the placenta (e.g. by the process of infarction or massive perivillous fibrin deposition) is based on subjective approximation done by examination of each slice of the placental disk. This method, although subjective, can give consistent results for a particular individual pathologist and has reasonable interobserver concordance.
6. Standardize the number and locations of sections of the placenta for histologic examination.
7. Standardize the gross and histologic descriptions of the placenta (see Appendix 1).
8. Familiarize yourself with the common gross and microscopic lesions (Tables 3 and 4) and specific placental abnormalities.
9. Consult for quick review and assessment the tables listing the salient features of the placenta in various maternal and fetal disorders (Tables 7 and 9).
10. In order to achieve consistency and specialization in reporting on placentas, it may be advisable to assign all placentas to one or two surgical pathologists within the group. I believe that taking such a systematic approach will lead to more intelligent and confident reporting on placentas without spending an undue amount of time and effort on the part of everyone concerned.

REFERENCES

1. Benirschke K: The placenta in the context of history and modern medical practice. *Arch Pathol Lab Med* 115:663–667, 1991.
2. Naeye R, Travers H: Report of the working group on the role of pathologist in malpractice litigation involving the placenta. *Arch Pathol Lab Med* 115:717–719, 1991.

3. Altshuler G: Placenta within the medicolegal imperative. *Arch Pathol Lab Med* 115:688–695, 1991.
4. Fox H: *Pathology of the placenta.* Saunders, Philadelphia, 1978.
5. Benirschke K, Kaufmann P: *Pathology of the human placenta*, 2nd ed. Springer-Verlag, New York, 1990.
6. Perrin EVDK: *Pathology of the placenta.* Churchill Livingstone, New York, 1984.
7. Fox H: Perivillous fibrin deposition in the human placenta. *Am J Obstet Gynecol* 98:245–251, 1967.
8. Burstein A, Berns AW, Hirata Y, et al: A comparative histologic and immunopathological study of the placenta in diabetes mellitus and in erythroblastosis fetalis. *Am J Obstet Gynecol* 86:66–76, 1963.
9. Driscoll SG: Placental examination in a clinical setting. *Arch Pathol Lab Med* 115:668–671, 1991.
10. Altshuler G: Indications for placental examination. *Arch Pathol Lab Med* 115:701–703, 1991.
11. Jauniaux E, Moscoso JG, Vanesse M, et al: Perfusion fixation for placental morphologic investigation. *Hum Pathol* 11:441–449, 1991.
12. Fox GE, Wesep RV, Resau JH, et al: The effect of immersion formaldehyde fixation on human placental weight. *Arch Pathol Lab Med* 115:726–728, 1991.
13. Altshuler G: The placenta. In *Diagnostic surgical pathology* (Sternberg SS, Ed). Raven Press, New York, 1989, p 1503.
14. Shanklin DR, Scott JS: Massive subchorial thrombohematoma (Brues' mole). *Br J Obstet Gynecol* 82:476–487, 1975.
15. Acker D, Sachs BP, Tracey KJ, et al: Abruptio placentae associated with cocaine use. *Am J Obstet Gynecol* 146:220–221, 1983.
16. Rushton DI: Placenta as a reflection of maternal disease, in *Pathology of placenta.* (Perrin, EDVK, Ed). Churchill Livingston. New York, 1984, p 70.
17. deSa DJ: Rupture of fetal vessels on placental surface. *Arch Dis Child* 46:495–501, 1971.
18. Shen-Schwarz S, Ruchelli E, Brown D: Villous edema of the placenta: A clinicopathologic study. *Placenta* 10:297–307, 1989.
19. Naeye RL, Maisel M, Loren J, et al: The clinical significance of placental villous edema. *Pediatrics* 71:588–594, 1983.
20. Altshuler G: Chorangiosis. An important placental sign of neonatal morbidity and mortality. *Arch Pathol Lab Med* 108:71–74, 1984.
21. Kaufmann P, Luckhardt M, Schweikhart G, et al: Cross sectional features and three-dimensional structure of human placental villi. *Placenta* 8:235–247, 1987.
22. Sander CH: Hemorrhagic endovasculitis and hemorrhagic villitis of the placenta. *Arch Pathol Lab Med* 104:371–373, 1980.
23. Sander CH, Kinnane L, Stevens NG, et al: Hemorrhagic endovasculitis of the placenta. A review with clinical correlation. *Placenta* 7:551–574, 1986.
24. Shen-Schwarz S, MacPherson TA, Mueller-Heubach E: The clinical significance of hemorrhagic endovasculitis of the placenta. *Obstet Gynecol* 65:637–641, 1985.
25. Silver MM, Yeger H, Lines LD: Hemorrhagic endovasculitis-like lesion induced in placental organ culture. *Hum Pathol* 19:251–256, 1988.
26. Robertson WB, Brosens I, Dixon HG: Uteroplacental vascular pathology. *Eur J Obstet Gynecol Reprod Biol* 5:47–65, 1975.
27. deWolf F, Robertson WB, Brosens I: The ultrastructure of acute atherosis in hypertensive pregnancy. *Am J Obstet Gynecol* 123:164–174, 1975.
28. Zeek PM, Assali NS: Vascular changes in the decidua associated with eclamptogenic toxemia of pregnancy. *Am J Clin Pathol* 20:1099–1109, 1950.

29. Reed GB, Clarieaux AE, Bain AD: *Disease of the fetus and newborn: Pathology, radiology and genetics*. Mosby, St. Louis, 1989, p 207.
30. Irving C, Hertiz AT: A study of placenta accreta. *Surg Gynecol Obstet* 64:178–200, 1937.
31. Naeye RL: Maternal floor infarction. *Hum Pathol* 16:823–828, 1985.
32. Robb JA, Benirschke K, Mannino F, et al: Intrauterine latent Herpes simplex virus infection. II. Latent neonatal infection. *Hum Pathol* 17:1210–1217, 1986.
33. Altshuler G, Russell P: The human placental villitides: A review of chronic intrauterine infection. *Curr Top Pathol* 60:64–112, 1975.
34. Jacques SM, Qureshi F: Chronic intervillositis of the placenta. *Arch Pathol Lab Med* 117:1032–1035, 1993.
35. Vawter GF: Perinatal listerosis. *Persp Pediatr Pathol* 6:153–166, 1981.
36. Fojaco RM, Hensley GT, Moskowitz L: Congenital syphilis and necrotizing funisitis. *JAMA* 261:1788–1790, 1989.
37. Naranbhai RC, Mathiassen W, Malan AF. Congenital tuberculosis localized to the ear. *Arch Dis Child* 64:738–740, 1989.
38. Kaplan C, Benirschke K, Tarzy B: Placental tuberculosis in early and late pregnancy. *Am J Obstet Gynecol* 137:858–860, 1980.
39. Dische MR, Quinn PA, Czegleay-Nagy E, et al: Genital mycoplasma infection: Intrauterine infection: Pathologic study of fetus and placenta. *Am J Clin Pathol* 72:167, 1979.
40. Fox H: Placental involvement in maternal systemic infection. *Persp Pediatr Pathol* 6:63–82, 1981.
41. Ornoy A, Segal S, Nishmi M, et al: Fetal and placental pathology in gestational rubella. *Am J Obstet Gynecol* 116:949–956, 1973.
42. Beecroft DMO: Prenatal cytomegalovirus infection: Epidemiology, pathology and pathogenesis. *Persp Pediatr Pathol* 6:203–242, 1981.
43. Garcia AGP: Fetal infection in chickenpox and alastrim with histopathologic study of the placenta. *Pediatrics* 32:895–901, 1963.
44. Singer DB: Pathology of neonatal Herpes simplex virus infection. *Persp Pediatr Pathol* 6:243–278, 1981.
45. Bendon RW, Perez F, Ray MB: Herpes simplex virus fetal and decidual infection. *Pediatr Pathol* 7:63–70, 1987.
46. Hyde SR, Giacoia GP: Congenital herpes infection: Placental and umbilical cord findings. *Obstet Gynecol* 81:852–855, 1993.
47. Schwartz DA, Caldwell E: Herpes simplex virus infection of the placenta. *Arch Pathol Lab Med* 115:1141–1144, 1991.
48. Ornoy A, Dudai M, Sadovsky E: Placental and fetal pathology in infectious mononucleosis: A possible indicator for Epstein–Barr virus teratogenicity. *Diagn Gynecol Obstet* 4:11–16, 1982.
49. Lucifora G, Calabro S, Carroccio G, et al: Immunocytochemical HBsAg evidence in the placentas of asymptomatic carrier mothers. *Am J Obstet Gynecol* 159:839–842, 1988.
50. Berry PJ, Gray ES, Porter HJ, et al: Parvovirus infection of the human fetus and newborn. *Semin Diagn Pathol* 9:4–12, 1992.
51. Knisely AS, O'Shea P, McMillan P, et al: Electron microscopic identification of parvovirus virions in erythroid-line cells in fatal hydrops fetalis. *Pediatr Pathol* 8:163–170, 1988.
52. Rogers BB, Mark Y, Oyer CE: Diagnosis and incidence of fetal parvovirus infection in an autopsy series. I: Histology. *Pediatr Pathol* 13:371–379, 1993.
53. Mark Y, Rogers BB, Oyer CE: Diagnosis and incidence of fetal parvovirus infection in an autopsy series. II: DNA amplification. *Pediatr Pathol* 13:381–386, 1993.

54. Joshi VV: Pathology of AIDS in children. Overview, update and future direction. Ann NY Acad Sci 693:71–92, 1993.
55. Jauniaux E, Nessmann C, Imbert MC, et al: Morphologic aspects of placenta in HIV pregnancies. Placenta 9:632–642, 1988.
56. Chandwani S, Greco MA, Mittal K, et al: Pathology and human immunodeficiency virus expression in placentas of seropositive women. J Inf Dis 163:1134–1138, 1991.
57. Martin AW, Brady K, Smith SI, et al: Immunohistochemical localization of HIV p24 antigen in placental tissue. Hum Pathol 23:411–414, 1992.
58. Maury W, Potts BJ, Robson AB: HIV-1 infection of first trimester and term human placental tissue. A possible mode of maternal fetal transmission. J Inf Dis 160:583–588, 1989.
59. Ehrnst A, Lindgren S, Dictor M, et al: HIV in pregnant women and their offspring: Evidence for late transmission. Lancet 388:203–207, 1991.
60. Bittencourt AL, dosSantos WLC, deOliviera CH: Placental and fetal candidiasis: Presentation of a case of an abortus. Mycopatholia 87:181–187, 1984.
61. VanBerger WS, Fleury FJ, Cheatle EL: Fatal maternal disseminated coccidioidomycosis in a nonendemic area. Am J Obstet Gynecol 124:661–664, 1976.
62. Kida M, Abramowsky CR, Santoscoy C: Cryptococcosis of the placenta in a woman with AIDS. Hum Pathol 20:920–921, 1989.
63. Bittencourt AL: Congenital Chagas' disease. Am J Dis Child 130:97–103, 1976.
64. Dische MR, Gooch WM: Congenital toxoplasmosis. Persp Pediatr Pathol 6:115–138, 1981.
65. Altshuler G: Placental villitis of unknown etiology: Harbinger of serious disease? A four months' experience of nine cases. J Reprod Med 11:215–222, 1973.
66. Khong TY, Staples A, Moore L, et al: Observer reliability in assessing villitis of unknown etiology. J Clin Pathol 46:208–210, 1993.
67. Russel P: Inflammatory lesions of the human placenta. III. The histology of villitis of unknown etiology. Placenta 1:227–244, 1980.
68. Redline RW, Abramowsky CR: Clinical and pathologic aspects of recurrent placental villitis. Hum Pathol 16:727–731, 1985.
69. Altshuler G: Placental infection and inflammation. In Pathology of the placenta (Perrin EVDK, Ed). Churchill Livingstone, New York, 1984, pp 141–163.
70. Labarre CA, McIntyre JA, Faulk WP: Immunohistologic evidence that villitis in human normal placentas is an immunologic lesion. Am J Obstet Gynecol 162:515–522, 1990.
70a. Redline RW, Patterson P. Villitis of unknown etiology is associated with major infiltration of fetal tissue by maternal inflammatory cells. Am J Pathol 143:473–479, 1993.
70b. Kliman MJ. The placenta revealed. Am J Pathol 143:332–336, 1993.
71. Kurman RJ: The morphology, biology, and pathology of intermediate trophoblast: A look back to the present. Hum Pathol 22:847–855, 1991.
72. Mazur MT, Kurman RJ: Gestational trophoblastic disease. In Blaustein's pathology of the female genital tract, 3rd ed (Kurman RJ, Ed). Springer-Verlag, New York, 1987, pp 835–875.
73. Fox H: Nontrophoblastic tumors of the placenta. In Pathology of the placenta (Perrin EVDK, Ed). Churchill Livingstone, New York, 1984, pp 199–210
74. Chen KTK, Ma CK, Kassel SH: Hepatocellular adenoma of the placenta. Am J Surg Pathol 10:436–440, 1986.
75. Naeye RL: Umbilical cord length: Clinical significance. J Pediatr 107:278–281, 1985.
76. deSa DJ: Diseases of the umbilical cord. In Pathology of the placenta (Perrin EVDK, Ed). Churchill Livingstone. New York, 1984, pp 121–139.

77. Kaplan C, Lowell DM, Salafia C: College of American Pathologists' Conference XIX on the examination of the placenta: Report of the working group on the definition of structural changes associated with abnormal function in the maternal/fetal/placental unit in the second and third trimesters. *Arch Pathol Lab Med* 115:709–716, 1991.

77a. Sander CM: Angiomatous malformation of placental chorionic stem vessels and pseudo-partial molar placentas: Report of five cases. *Pediatr Pathol* 13:621–633, 1993.

78. Khong Ty, Dilly SA: Calcification of umbilical artery: two distinct lesions. *J Clin Pathol* 42:931–934, 1989.

79. Hovatta O, Lipasti A, Rapola J, et al: Causes of stillbirth: A clinicopathologic study of 243 patients. *Br J Obstet Gynecol* 90:691–695, 1983.

80. Browne FJ: On abnormalities of umbilical cord which may cause antenatal death. *J Obstet Gynecol Br Emp* 32:17–48, 1925.

81. Edmonds HW: The spiral twist of the normal umbilical cord in twin and in singletons. *Am J Obstet Gynecol* 67:102–120, 1954.

82. Robertson RD, Rubinstein LM, Wolfson WL, et al: Constriction of the umbilical cord as a cause of fetal demise following midtrimester amniocentesis. *J Reprod Med* 26:325–327, 1981.

83. Coulter JBS, Scott JM, Jordan MM: Edema of the cord and respiratory distress in the newborn. *Br J Obstet Gynecol* 82:453–459, 1975.

84. Jauniaux E, Munter CD, Vanesse M, et al: Embryonic remnants of the umbilical cord: Morphologic and clinical aspects. *Hum Pathol* 20:458–462, 1989.

85. Blanc WA, Allan GW: Intrafunicular ulceration of persistent omphalomesenteric duct with intra-amniotic hemorrhage and fetal death. *Am J Obstet Gynecol* 72:1392–1396, 1961.

86. Heifetz SA, Reuda-Pedraz ME: Hemangiomas of the umbilical cord. *Pediatr Pathol* 1:385–389, 1983.

86a. Levy H, Meier PR, Madkowski EL. Umbilical cord prolapse. *Obstet Gynecol* 64:499–502, 1984.

87. Landing BH. Amnion nodosum: A lesion of the placenta apparently associated with deficient secretion of urine. *Am J Obstet Gynecol* 60:1339–1342, 1950.

88. Torpin R: *Fetal malformation caused by amnion rupture during gestation.* Charles C Thomas, Springfield, IL, 1968.

89. Heifetz SA: Strangulation of the umbilical cord by amniotic bands. Report of 6 cases and literature review. *Pediatr Pathol* 2:285–304, 1984.

90. Young ID, Lindenbaum RH, Thompson EM, et al: Amniotic bands in connective tissue disorders. *Arch Dis Child* 60:1061–1063, 1985.

91. Lockwood L, Ghidini A, Romero R, et al: Amniotic band syndrome: Re-evaluation of its pathogenesis. *Am J Obstet Gynecol* 160:1030–1033, 1989.

92. Mahony BS, Filly RA, Callen PW, et al: The amniotic band syndrome: Antenatal sonographic diagnosis and potential pitfalls. *Am J Obstet Gynecol* 152:63–68, 1985.

93. Falciglia HS, Kosmetatos N, Brady K, et al: Intrauterine meconium aspiration in an extremely premature infant. *Am J Dis Child* 147:1035–1037, 1993.

94. Katz VL, Bowes WA: Meconium aspiration syndrome: Reflections on a murky subject. *Am J Obstet Gynecol* 166:171–183, 1992.

95. Wiswell TE, Bent RC: Meconium staining and the meconium aspiration syndrome. Unresolved issues. *Pediatr Clin North Am* 40:955–981, 1993.

96. Cunningham FG, MacDonald PC, Gant NF: *Williams' obstetrics.* Appleton & Lange. Norwalk, CT, 1989, Chap 31, p 553.

97. Fujikura T, Klionsky B: The significance of meconium staining. *Am J Obstet Gynecol* 121:45–50, 1975.

98. Miller PW, Coen RW, Benirschke K: Dating the time interval from meconium passage to birth. *Obstet Gynecol* 66:459–462, 1985.
99. McPherson T: Fact or fancy. What can we really tell from the placenta. *Arch Pathol Lab Med* 115:672–681, 1991.
100. Altshuler G, Hyde S: Meconium-induced vasoconstriction: A potential cause of cerebral and other fetal hypoperfusion and of poor frequency outcome. *J Child Neurol* 4:137–142, 1989.
101. Naeye RL: Functionally important disorders of the placenta, umbilical cord and fetal membranes. *Hum Pathol* 18:680–691, 1987.
102. Altshuler G: Placental infection and inflammation. In *Pathology of the placenta* (Perrin EVDK, Ed). Churchill Livingstone, New York, 1984, pp 141–163.
103. Lauweryns J, Bernat R, Lerut A, et al: Intrauterine pneumonia. *Biol Neonate* 22:301–318, 1973.
104. deSa DJ: Infection and amniotic aspiration of middle ear in stillbirths and neonatal deaths. *Arch Dis Child* 48:872–880, 1973.
105. Hillier SL, Martius J, Krohn M, et al: A case control study of chorioamnionic infection and histologic chorioamnionitis in prematurity. *N Engl J Med* 319:972–978, 1988.
106. Schlievert P, Larsen B, Johnson W, et al: Bacterial growth inhibition by amniotic fluid. *Am J Obstet Gynecol* 122:809–819, 1975.
107. Lamont RF, Fisk N: The role of infection in the pathogenesis of preterm labour. *Progr Obstet Gynecol* 10:135–158, 1993.
108. Gersell DJ, Phillips NJ, Beckerman K: Chronic chorioamnionitis: A clinicopathologic study of 17 cases. *Int J Gynecol Pathol* 10:217–229, 1991.
109. Gersell DJ: Chronic villitis, chronic chorioamnionitis and maternal floor infarction. *Semin Diagn Pathol* 10:251–256, 1993.
110. Benirschke K: Congenital syphilis and necrotizing funisitis. *JAMA* 262:904, 1989.
111. Hood IC, DeSa DJ, White RK: The inflammatory response in candidal chorioamnionitis. *Hum Pathol* 14:984–990, 1983.
112. DeWolf F, Brosens I, Renaer M: Fetal growth retardation and maternal arterial supply of the human placenta in the absence of sustained hypertension. *Br J Obstet Gynecol* 87:678–685, 1980.
113. Kitzmiller JS, Watt N, Driscoll SG: Decidual arteriopathy in hypertension and diabetes in pregnancy: Immunofluorescent studies. *Am J Obstet Gynecol* 141:773–779, 1981.
114. Weinstein L: Preeclampsia/eclampsia with hemolysis, elevated liver enzymes, and thrombocytopenia: *Obstet Gynecol* 66:657–660, 1985.
115. Singer DB: The placenta in pregnancies complicated by diabetes mellitus. *Persp Pediat Pathol* 8:199–212.
116. Teasdale F: Histomorphometry of the human class C diabetes mellitus. *Placenta* 5:69–86, 1984.
117. Jones CJP, Fox H: Placental changes in gestational diabetes: An ultrastructural study. *Obstet Gynecol* 48:274–280, 1976.
118. Lage JM, Popek EJ: The role of DNA flow cytometry in evaluation of partial and complete hydatidiform moles and hydropic abortions. *Semin Diagn Pathol* 10:267–274, 1993.
119. Howat AJ, Beck S, Fox H, et al: Can histopathologists reliably diagnose molar pregnancy? *J Clin Pathol* 46:599–602, 1993.
119a. Rushton DI: Examination of products of conception from previable human pregnancies. *J Clin Pathol* 34:819–835, 1981.
119b. Novak RW, Malone JM, Robinson HB: The role of the pathologist in the evaluation of first trimester abortions. *Pathol Annu* 25:297–311, 1990.

119c. Fox H: Histological classification of tissue from spontaneous abortions: A valueless exercise? *Histopathology* 22:599–600, 1993.
120. Conran RM, Hitchcock CL, Popek EJ, et al: Diagnostic considerations in molar gestation. *Hum Pathol* 24:41–48, 1993.
121. Lage JM, Mark SD, Robert DJ, et al: A flow cytometric study of 137 fresh hydropic placentas: Correlation between types of hydatidiform mole and nuclear DNA ploidy. *Obstet Gynecol* 79:403–410, 1992.
122. Aladjem S: Placenta of premature infant. *Am J Obstet Gynecol* 102:311–312, 1968.
123. Toth M, Witkin SS, Ledger W, et al: The role of infection in the etiology of preterm birth. *Obstet Gynecol* 71:723–736, 1988.
124. Baldwin VJ, MacLeod PM, Benirschke K: Placental findings in alcohol abuse in pregnancy. *Birth Defects* 18:89–94, 1982.
125. Asmussen I: Ultrastructure of the villi and fetal capillaries in placentas from smoking and non-smoking mothers. *Br J Obstet Gynecol* 87:239–245, 1980.
126. Teasdale F, Ghislaine JJ: Morphological changes in the placentas of smoking mothers: A histomorphometric study. *Biol Neonate* 55:251–259, 1989.
127. Mastrogiannis DS, Decavalas GO, Verma V, et al: Perinatal outcome after recurrent cocaine usage. *Obstet Gynecol* 76:8–11, 1990.
128. Naeye RL, Blanc W, Leblanc W, et al: Fetal complications of maternal heroin addiction: Abnormal growth, infections and episodes of stress. *J Pediatr* 83:1055–1061, 1973.
129. Abramowsky CR, Vegas ME, Swinehart G, et al: Decidual vasculopathy of the placenta in lupus erythematosus. *N Engl J Med* 303:668–672, 1980.
130. Branch DW, Scott JR, Kochenour NK, et al: Obstetric complications associated with lupus anticoagulant. *N Engl J Med* 313:1322–1326, 1985.
131. Robertson EG, Neer KJ: Placental injection studies in twin gestation. *Am J Obstet* 147:170–174, 1983.
132. Strong SJ, Corney G: *The placenta in twin pregnancy*. Pergamon Press, Oxford (UK), 1967, pp 65–77.
133. Blickstein I: The twin-twin transfusion syndrome. *Obstet Gynecol* 76:714–722, 1990.
134. Klebe JG, Ingomar CJ: The fetoplacental circulation during parturition illustrated by interfetal transfusion syndrome. *Pediatrics* 49:112–115, 1972.
135. Bendon RW, Siddiqui T: Acute twin-twin in utero transfusion. *Pediatr Pathol* 9:591–598, 1989.
136. Benirschke K: Intrauterine death of a twin: Mechanisms, implications for surviving twin, and placental pathology. *Semin Diagn Pathol* 10:222–231, 1993.
137. Grafe MR: Antenatal cerebral necrosis in monochorionic twins. *Pediatr Pathol* 13:15–19, 1993.
138. Benirschke K: Twin placenta in perinatal mortality. *NY State J Med* 61:1499–1508, 1961.
139. Lage JM, Vanmarter LJ, Mikhail E: Vascular anastomoses in fused, dichorionic twin placentas resulting in twin transfusion syndrome. *Placenta* 10:55–59, 1989.
140. Levi S: Ultrasonic assessment of the high rate of human multiple pregnancy in the first trimester. *J Clin Ultrasound* 4:3–5, 1976.
141. Jauniaux E, Elkazen N, Leroy F, et al: Clinical and morphologic aspects of vanishing twin phenomenon. *Obstet Gynecol* 72:577–581, 1988.
142. Harper RG, Kenigsburg K, Sia CG, et al: Xiphopagus conjoined twins: A 300-year review of the obstetric, morphopathologic, neonatal and surgical parameters. *Am J Obstet Gynecol* 137:617–629, 1980.
143. Potter EL, Craig JM: *Pathology of the fetus and infant*, 3rd ed. Year Book Medical Publishers, Chicago, 1975. pp 226–233.
144. Machin GA: Hydrops revisited: Literature review of 1414 cases published in 1980s. *Am J Med Genet* 34:366–390, 1989.

145. Popek E: *The placenta in fetal disorders.* Syllabus of the course on placental pathology sponsored by Armed Forces Institute of Pathology, October 24, 1991, Washington, DC.
146. Jones CJP, Mehroo L, Chawner LE, et al: Ultrastructure of the human placenta in metabolic storage disease. *Placenta* 11:395–411, 1990.
147. Hug G, Soukop S, Ryan M, et al: Rapid prenatal diagnosis of glycogen storage type II by electron microscopy of uncultured amniotic cells. *N Engl J Med* 310:1018–1022, 1984.
148. Kalousek DK: Confined placental mosaicism. *Pediatr Pathol* 10:69–72, 1990.
149. Johnson A, Wapner RJ, Davis GH, et al: Mosaicism in chorionic villous sampling: An association with poor perinatal outcome. *Obstet Gynecol* 75:573–576, 1990.
150. Genest DR: Estimating the time of death in stillborn fetuses: II. Histologic evaluation of the placenta; a study of 71 stillborns. *Obstet Gynecol* 80:585–592, 1992.
151. Jauniaux E, Donner C, Simon P, et al: Pathologic aspects of umbilical cord after percutaneous umbilical blood sampling. *Obstet Gynecol* 73:215–218, 1989.
152. Williams JK, McCalin L, Rosemurgy AS, et al: Evaluation of blunt abdominal trauma in the third trimester of pregnancy. *Obstet Gynecol* 75:33–37, 1990.
153. Gavriil P, Jauniaux E, Leroy F: Pathologic examination of placentas from singleton and twin pregnancies obtained after in vitro fertilization and embryo transfer. *Pediatr Pathol* 13:453–462, 1993.
154. De Lia JE, Kuhlmann RS, Cruikshank DP, et al: Current topic: Placental surgery: A new frontier. *Placenta* 14:477–485, 1993.
155. De Lia JE, Cruikshank DP, Keye WR Jr: Fetoscopic neodymium-YAG laser occlusion of placental vessels in severe twin-twin transfusion syndrome. *Obstet Gynecol* 75:1046–1053, 1990.

INDEX

A
Abnormalities of placenta
  gross abnormalities, 22–32
    fetal blood flow, lesions due to
        disturbance of, 29–30
      fetal artery thrombosis, 30
      intervillous thrombus, 29
      Kline's hemorrhage, 29–30
      subamniotic hematoma, 30
    maternal blood flow, lesions due to
        disturbance of, 22–29
      marginal hematoma, 28
      perivillous fibrin, 22–24
      placental infarct, 28–29
      retroplacental hematoma, 25–28
      subchorionic fibrin, 24
      subchorionic thrombosis, 24–25
    noncirculatory lesions, 30–32
      calcification, 30–31
      chorionic cyst, 31–32
  histologic lesions, 32–41
    basement membrane, 34–35
    cytotrophoblastic cells, excessive
        number of, 33
    fetal stem arteries, 37–41
      fibromuscular sclerosis, 37
      hemorrhagic endovasculitis, 38
      obliterative endarteritis, 37–38
    fibrinoid necrosis of villi, 34
    intravillous fibrinoid, 34
    maternal uteroplacental arteries,
        histopathology of, 38–41
    placental villi, 32–37
    stromal abnormality, 35–36
      Hofbauer cells, excessive number
          of, 36
      stromal fibrosis, 35
      villous edema, 35–36
    syncytial knots, excessive number of,
        32–33
    trophoblast abnormality, 32–37
    vasculosyncytial membrane, 34
    villus
      blood vessel abnormality, 36
      generalized abnormality of, 36–37
        accelerated maturation, 37
        villous immaturity, 36
Abortion, 85, 88–89
Abruptio placentae, 45, 87, 92
Acardiac twin, 95, 107–108
Accelerated maturation, villus, 37
Accessory lobe, with placenta, 43
Alcohol abuse, placental features, 87,
    91–92
Amnion
  cyst, 69
  extraamniotic pregnancy, 72
  lesions of, 67–81
  nodosum, 68–69
  polyp, 69
  rest, 69
  web, 69
Amniotic band syndrome, 70–71
Amniotic fluid
  embolism, 80–81
  human immunodeficiency virus, 55
Aneurysm, umbilical cord, 61–62
Antepartum intrauterine death, lesions of
    placenta, 97, 111–112
Anticardiolipin, placental features, 87,
    92

B
Bacterial villitis, 49–51
  Chlamydia infection, 51
  Listeria monocytogenes, 50–51
  Mycobacterium tuberculosis, 51
  Mycoplasma infection, 51
  Syphilis, congenital, 51
  Treponema pallidum, 51
Barrier, placental, human
    immunodeficiency virus, 56
Basal place, histologic assessment, 21
Basement membrane, 34–35
  trophoblastic, 34–35
Bilobate placenta, 43
Blood vessels, umbilical cord
  calcification, 63

Blood vessels, umbilical cord (*contd.*)
  hematoma, 62–63
  thrombosis, 62
Brues's mole, 24–25

C
Calcification, 30–31
  umbilical blood vessel, 63
Chlamydial infection, 51
Chorioamnionitis
  acute, 75–80
  chronic, 80
Chorion
  cyst, 31–32
  lesions of, 67–81
  plate, histologic assessment, 20
Chromosomal disorders, lesions of placenta, 96, 110
Cigarette abuse, placental features, 87, 91–92
Cocaine abuse, placental features, 87, 91–92
Conjoined twins, 108
Coxsackie virus, villitis, 52
Cyst
  amnion, 69
  chorion, 31–32
  umbilical cord, 66
Cytomegalovirus, villitis, 51–52
Cytotrophoblastic cells, excessive number of, 33

D
Decidua, 81
Decidual vasculopathy, 81
Deciduitis, 81
Delivery, premature, placental features, 86, 89–90
Development of placenta, 2
Diabetes, maternal, 84–85
Dichorionic diamniotic placenta, 93, 106

E
Echo virus, villitis, 52
Edema
  umbilical cord, 65
  villus, 35–36
Embolism, amniotic fluid, 80–81
Embryonic remnants, of umbilical cord, 66
Embryo transfer, placenta in, 113
Endarteritis, obliterative, 37–38

Endovasculitis, hemorrhagic, 38
Entanglement, umbilical cord, 67
Erythroblastosis fetalis, lesions of placenta, 95, 109
Examination of placenta, in clinical setting, 12–13
Extraamniotic pregnancy, 72
Extrachorial placentas, 42–43
Extramembranous pregnancy, 71–72

F
Fetal blood flow, lesions due to disturbance, 29–30
  fetal artery thrombosis, 30
  intervillous thrombus, 29
  Kline's hemorrhage, 29–30
  subamniotic hematoma, 30
Fetal disorders
  acardiac twin, 95, 107–108
  antepartum intrauterine death, 97, 111–112
  artery thrombosis, 30
  blood flow disturbance, 29–30
  chromosomal disorder, 96, 110
  conjoined twins, 108
  dichorionic diamniotic placenta, 93, 106
  erythroblastosis fetalis, 95, 109
  fetus compressus, 94, 107
  fetus papyraceous, 94, 107
  human immunodeficiency virus, 55–56
  intrapartum fetal death, 112
  intrauterine growth retardation, 95, 109
  lesions of placenta, 92–112
  metabolic disorders, 96, 110
  monochorionic diamniotic placenta, 93, 104–106
  monochorionic monoamniotic placenta, 94, 106–107
  multiple birth, lesions of placenta, 92–108
  nonimmunologic hydrops fetalis, 96, 110
  triplet birth, lesions of placenta, 108
  twin birth, lesions of placenta, 92–108
  vanishing twins, 94, 107
Fetal stem arteries, 37–41
  fibromuscular sclerosis, 37
  hemorrhagic endovasculitis, 38
  histologic assessment, 20
  obliterative endarteritis, 37–38

Fever, maternal, placental features, 87, 91
Fibrin
    intravillous, 34
    perivillous, 22–24
    in placenta, 2–12
    subchorionic, 24
Fibrosis, stromal, of villi 35, 47–48
Fungal infection, 56
Funisitis, 80
    umbilical cord, 67

G

Genital tract, maternal, human immunodeficiency virus, 54
Granulomatous villitis, 47
Gross examination, of placenta, 14–22
Growth retardation, intrauterine, lesions of placenta, 95, 109

H

Hemangioma, placenta, 59
Hematoma
    marginal, 28
    retroplacental, 25–28
    subamniotic, 30
    umbilical blood vessel, 62–63
Hemorrhage, Kline's, 29–30
Hemorrhagic endovasculitis, 38
Hepatitis virus, 53
Heroin abuse, placental features, 87, 91–92
Herpes simplex, viral villitis, 52
Histologic examination, of placenta, 16–22
Histologic lesions
    basement membrane, 34–35
    cytotrophoblastic cell, excessive number of, 33
    fetal stem arteries, 37–41
        fibromuscular sclerosis, 37
        hemorrhagic endovasculitis, 38
        obliterative endarteritis, 37–38
    fibrinoid necrosis of villus, 34
    intravillous fibrinoid, 34
    maternal uteroplacental artery, histopathology of, 38–41
    placenta, 32–41
    stromal abnormality, 35–36
        Hofbauer cells, excessive number of, 36
        stromal fibrosis, 35
    villous edema, 35–36
    trophoblast abnormality, 32–37
    vasculosyncytial membrane, 34
    villus, 32–37
        blood vessel abnormality, 36
        generalized abnormality of, 36–37
            accelerated maturation, 37
            villous immaturity, 36
        syncytial knots, excessive number of, 32–33
Hofbauer cells, excessive number of, 36
Human immunodeficiency virus
    amniotic fluid, 55
    fetal tissue, 55
        maternal genital tract, 54
        placenta, 54–55
    placental barrier, 56
Human parvovirus, viral villitis, 53
Hydrops fetalis, nonimmunologic, lesions of placenta, 96, 110
Hypertension, maternal, 84, 85

I

Iatrogenic lesions, placenta, 112–113
Immature villi, 36
    intermediate, structure, 17
    Infarct, placental, 28–29
    Insertion, abnormal, umbilical cord, 63
    Intermediate villi, structure, 17
    Intervillositis, chronic, 48–49
    Intervillous space, histologic assessment, 20
    Intervillous thrombus, 29
    Intrapartum fetal death, lesions of placenta, 112
    Intrauterine death, antepartum, lesions of placenta, 97, 111–112
    Intrauterine growth retardation, lesions of placenta, 95, 109
    Intravillous fibrinoid, 34
    In vitro fertilization, placenta in, 113

K

Kline's hemorrhage, 29–30
Knot(s)
    syncytial, excessive number of, 32–33
    umbilical cord, 63–64

L

Labor, premature, placental features, 86, 89–90
Large placenta, 41–42

Laser surgery, 113–114
Listeria monocytogenes, bacterial villitis, 50–51
Lobe
  accessory, 43
  bilobate placenta, 43
  succenturiate, 43
Long umbilical cord, 61–62
Lupus anticoagulant, placental features, 87, 92

M

Marginal hematoma, 28
Maternal blood flow, lesions due to disturbance of, 22–29
  marginal hematoma, 28
  perivillous fibrin, 22–24
  placental infarct, 28–29
  retroplacental hematoma, 25–28
  subchorionic fibrin, 24
  subchorionic thrombosis, 24–25
Maternal disorders
  abortion, 85, 88–89
  abruptio placentae, 87, 92
  anticardiolipin, 87, 92
  blood flow disturbance, 22–29
  diabetes, 84–85
  fever, placental features, 87, 91
  floor infarction, 45–46
  genital tract, human immunodeficiency virus, 54
  hypertension, 84, 85
  lesions of placenta in, 81–92
  lupus anticoagulant, 87, 92
  maternal fever, 87, 91
  oligohydramnios, 86, 90–91
  polyhydramnios, 86, 90–91
  postmaturity, 86, 90
  premature labor/delivery, 86, 89–90
  substance abuse, 87, 91–92
  systemic lupus erythematosus, 87, 92
  toxemia, 81–83, 85
Maternal uteroplacental arteries, histopathology of, 38–41
Maturation, villus
  accelerated, 37
Meconium staining, of membrane, 72–75
Membranes
  amnion nodosum, 68–69
  amniotic band syndrome, 70–71
  amniotic cyst, 69
  amniotic fluid embolism, 80–81
  amniotic polyp, 69
  amniotic rest, 69
  amniotic web, 69
  chorioamnionitis
    acute, 75–80
    chronic, 80
  extraamniotic pregnancy, 72
  extramembranous pregnancy, 71–72
  funisitis, 80
  histologic assessment, 21
  iatrogenic lesions, 112–113
  lesions of, 67–81
  meconium staining of, 72–75
  rupture of, 86, 91
  squamous metaplasia, 68
  tumors of, 81
Mesenchymal villi, structure, 17
Metabolic disorders, lesions of placenta, 96, 110
Metaplasia, squamous, membrane, 68
Metastic tumors, placenta, 60
Mole, Brues's, 24–25
Monochorionic diamniotic placenta, 93, 104–106
Monochorionic monoamniotic placenta, 94, 106–107
Mononucleosis, viral villitis, 52
Multiple birth, lesions of placenta, 92–108
Mycobacterium tuberculosis, bacterial villitis, 51
Mycoplasma infection, bacterial villitis, 51

N

Necrotizing villitis, 47
Noncirculatory lesions, 30–32
  calcification, 30–31
  chorionic cyst, 31–32
Nonimmunologic hydrops fetalis, lesions of placenta, 96, 110

O

Obliterative endarteritis, 37–38
Oligohydramnios, placental features, 86, 90–91

P

Parasitic infection, 56–57
Parvovirus, human, 53
Pathologic examination
  gross examination, 14–22

histologic examination, 16–22
indications for, 14
procedure, 14–22
Pathologist, clinical data sent to, 13–14
Perivillous fibrin, 22–24
Placenta
  decidua, see Decidua
  Laser surgery, 113–114
  membrane, see Membrane
  umbilical cord, see Umbilical cord
Placenta accreta, 44–45
Placenta membranacea, 43
Placenta previa, 43–44
Poliomyelitis, 53
Polyhydramnios, placental features, 86, 90–91
Polyp, amnion, 69
Postmaturity, placental features, 86, 90
Premature labor/delivery, 86, 89–90
Premature rupture, of membrane, 86, 91
Preterm rupture, of membrane, 86, 91
Prolapse, umbilical cord, 67
Proliferative villitis, 47
Prolonged rupture, of membrane, 86, 91

R
Remnant, embryonic, of umbilical cord, 66
Reparative villitis, 47
Rest, amnion, 69
Retroplacental hematoma, 25–28, 45
Rubella, viral villitis, 51–52
Rupture
  of membrane, 86, 91
  of umbilical blood vessel, 62–63

S
Sclerosis, fibromuscular, 37
Short umbilical cord, 61–62
Siamese twins, see Conjoined twins
Small placenta, 42
Specimen, retention of, 22
Squamous metaplasia, membrane, 68
Staining, meconium, of membrane, 72–75
Stem villus, structure, 17
Stricture, umbilical cord, 64–65
Stromal abnormality, 35–36
  fibrosis, 35, 47–48
  Hofbauer cells, excessive number of, 36
  stromal fibrosis, 35

villous edema, 35–36
Structure of placenta, 2–12
Subamniotic hematoma, 30
Subchorial thrombosis, 24–25
Subchorionic fibrin, 24
Subchorionic thrombosis, 24–25
Substance abuse, placental features, 87, 91–92
Succenturiate lobe, 43
Surgical pathology report, 22
Syncytial knots, excessive number of, 32–33
Syphilis, congenital, bacterial villitis, 51
Systemic lupus erythematous, placental features, 87, 92

T
Teratoma
  of placenta, 59–60
  of placental membranes, 81
Terminal villi, structure, 17
Thrombosis, fetal artery, 30
Thrombus, intervillous, 29
Tobacco abuse, placental features, 87, 91–92
Torsion, umbilical cord, 64
Toxemia, 81–83, 85
Transfusion syndrome, twin
  neonatal criteria for diagnosis, 105
  ultrasound criteria, 105
Traumatic lesions placenta, 113
Treponema pallidum, bacterial villitis, 51
Triplet birth, lesions of placenta, 108
Trisomy, lesions of placenta, 96, 110
Trophoblast abnormalities, 32–37
Tumors
  membranes, 81
  placenta, 58–60
  umbilical cord, 66–67
Twin
  acardiac, 95, 107–108
  birth, lesions of placenta, 92–108
  conjoined, 108
  transfusion syndrome
    Laser surgery, 113–114
    neonatal criteria for diagnosis, 105
    ultrasound criteria, 105
  vanishing, 94, 107

U
Ultrasound criteria, twin transfusion syndrome, 105

Umbilical cord
  abnormal insertion of, 63
  aneurysm, 61–62
  blood vessel
    calcification, 63
    hematoma, 62–63
    rupture, 62–63
    thrombosis, 62
  cyst, 66
  edema, 65
  embryonic remnants of, 66
  entanglement, 67
  funisitis, 67
  histologic assessment, 21
  iatrogenic lesions, 112–113
  knot, 63–64
  lesions of, 60–67
  long, 61–62
  prolapse, 67
  short, 61–62
  single umbilical artery, 61
  stricture, 64–65
  supernumerary umbilical vessels, 61
  torsion, 64
  tumor, 66–67
  varix, 61–62
  vasculitis, 67
Uteroplacental arteries, maternal, histopathology of, 38–41

V

Vaccinia, viral villitis, 52
Vanishing twins, 94, 107
Varicella, viral villitis, 52
Variola minor, viral villitis, 52
Varix, umbilical cord, 61–62
Vasculitis, umbilical cord, 67
Vasculopathy, decidual, 81
Vasculosyncytial membrane, 34
Vessels, supernumerary, umbilical, 61
Villitis, 46–58
  bacterial, 49–51
    chlamydia infection, 51
    Listeria monocytogenes, 50–51
    Mycobacterium tuberculosis, 51
    Mycoplasma infection, 51
    Syphilis, congenital, 51
    Treponema pallidum, 51
  fungal infection, 56
  intervillositis, chronic, 48–49
  parasitic infection, 56–57
  unknown etiology, 57–58
  viral, 51–54
    Coxsackie virus, 52
    cytomegalovirus, 51–52
    Echovirus, 52
    hepatitis virus, 53
    herpes simplex, 52
    human immunodeficiency virus, 54–56
    human parvovirus, 53
    mononucleosis, 52
    poliomyelitis, 53
    rubella, 51–52
    vaccinia, 52
    varicella, 52
    variola minor, 52
Villus
  accelerated maturation, 37
  blood vessel abnormality, 36
  edema, 35–36
  fibrinoid necrosis of, 34
  generalized abnormality of, 36–37
    accelerated maturation, 37
    villous immaturity, 36
  immaturity, 36
  placental, 32–37
  structure, 16–20
Viral villitis, 51–54
  Coxsackie virus, 52
  cytomegalovirus, 51–52
  Echovirus, 52
  hepatitis virus, 53
  herpes simplex, 52
  human immunodeficiency virus, 54–56
  human parvovirus, 53
  mononucleosis, 52
  poliomyelitis, 53
  rubella, 51–52
  vaccinia, 52
  varicella, 52
  variola minor, 52

W

Web, amniotic, 69